The Golden Thread

A quiet revolution in holistic cancer care

Pat Pilkington, MBE

First published in 2015 by Vala Publishing Co-operative

Vala Publishing Co-operative Ltd
8 Gladstone Street, Bristol, BS3 3AY, UK

For further information on Vala publications, see
www.valapublishers.coop or write to info@valapublishers.coop

Cover artwork by Sue Gent
www.suegentdesign.com

Typeset in Freya
Printed and bound by CPI Antony Rowe, Chippenham, UK
The paper used is Munken Premium, which is FSC certified.

This book was written by the late Pat Pilkington but edited and published after her death. Every effort has been made to check dates and references within the text, but the publisher apologises for any inaccuracies, and will endeavour to put them right in any future editions of the book.

A CIP catalogue record for this title is available from the British Library.

ISBN 978-1-908363-12-1

To Tim Tiley, without whom none
of this would have happened

Contents

Introduction by Penny Brohn Cancer Care

Pat Pilkington dedicated thirty-four years of her life to our charity, which she founded with her dear friend Penny Brohn when Penny was first diagnosed with cancer in 1979.

This book explores her unique spiritual vision and tells of the care that she personally provided to those affected by cancer and their loved ones up until the month of her own death in August 2013.

Within the pages of this book she weaves the story of the history of the centre with her personal quest for the spiritual 'Golden Thread' that enthralled both Pat and her beloved husband Christopher. Pat married Christopher in 1954 and began what she described as 'life as an ordinary vicar's wife': a life that was to become anything but ordinary. Pat and Penny pioneered the 'Whole Person Approach' that is at the core of the work of the charity today, however in this book she shines a spotlight in particular on her own spiritual journey.

Our vision today at Penny Brohn is to provide life-changing, whole person support to everyone affected by cancer. We see every person as a whole, made up of mind, body, spirit and emotions. We respect each person and their differences and this includes respecting different approaches to spirituality and those who have no faith. This was also reflected in Pat's own working practice, she did not care what the person in need believed in – she reached out from a position of compassion to meet them where they were. We continue to work with these values at the core of our approach.

Our unique combination of courses, tools and techniques includes lifestyle measures such as healthy eating, physical activity, ways of managing stress and emotions, supporting your spirit and a range of complementary therapies. Our programme is designed to work alongside medical and other cancer treatments and to be a useful and integrated resource for people in their journey with cancer. The services offered free by the charity are explained in full after Pat's story, on page 147.

Pat and Penny's influence continues to frame the discussion and enquiries that underpin our services and keep us rooted in our history and the original vision of the charity: that all people affected by cancer get the support they need to live as well as they can.

This book offers an opportunity to discover how the charity came into being and to explore with Pat her spiritual path – a tangible golden thread that shone through every aspect of this inspirational woman's life.

Michael Connors, Director of Services at Penny Brohn Cancer Care

Foreword by Caroline Myss

I've been asked to write many book forewords throughout my career, but none for a dear and remarkable friend who was dying as I wrote. Were it not for the fact that Pat told me that she was ready to 'go home' and that she knew she would be with her beloved late husband, Christopher, I would have been too shattered to undertake this task. Even as Pat said those words to me, I remembered that Christopher had told her the same thing just as he entered the early stages of his own terminal illness. Entering the final stages of one's life consciously, no less cheerfully, may well be the most remarkable testimony to a life fully lived in the power of love and grace.

There are so many wonderful things that I can say about Pat, but I will begin with this fact: Pat Pilkington lived a life that is worthy of being remembered as well as being studied. Pat became a Sage, a Mystic, and a Healer. She never stopped refining her inner spiritual resources, always polishing her perceptions of love, life, God, and evolving humanity.

As someone who has been in the publishing, editing, and writing field for over thirty years, I can tell you that all memoirs are not alike. That is, when a person settles into the formidable challenge of recording his or her life's story, that individual has to organize a selection of facts and events. What is the story about their life they wish to tell? Some people want to record their adventures and others their trials and tribulations, or their love affairs. Few people, in other words, can include every single detail.

A theme, a golden thread, must be chosen around which the individual gathers specific memories, events, and dates in order to relay the one significant message for which they want to be remembered.

The theme of Pat's life – her golden thread – has always been one of service to humanity and the refinement of love, faith, and spiritual truth. In fact, she had no choice but to write a spiritual memoir. The same can be said of Christopher. Their marriage was a true union of heart, mind, and soul threaded together. Every one who met them in some way was blessed, whether they knew them for a day or for years. Pat's constant focus was, "What do I need to do? How can I help? What needs to be done? Who needs attention?"

Their life story was also an illustration of how faith and love move mountains to cooperate with human effort. Mind you, I did not say that faith and love made things easy but Pat and Christopher somehow knew how to cooperate with the will of the Divine. The power of faith and love are the interwoven themes that Pat chose as the threads of her memoir, though I honestly do not believe she consciously intended for that theme to present itself. Rather, while Pat is describing one event or one challenge, she writes so confidently about love and the nature of the spirit that her life and her wisdom seem to be one and the same thing. Somehow, she has managed to communicate the power of love and her profound beliefs in a way that only inspires. And, although devoted to the Christian path, Pat was simultaneously genuinely accepting of the truth in all other spiritual traditions. I have rarely met a human being who so lived the message of, "Love one another as I have loved you". If it can be said that a person can breathe love, then such was true about Pat.

She has left many, many legacies behind, among them the Penny Brohn Cancer Care charity. I met Pat because of the Centre, which I consider to be one of the most impressive health facilities

I have ever had the pleasure to be associated with.

I consider this superb book, *The Golden Thread*, to be yet another of Pat's great accomplishments as it is a compilation of a remarkable woman's spiritual journey and how she truly lived the message of love. Pat's life illustrates that a human being can live the spiritual life fully and not be denied any expression of love, as so many people fear.

It is my hope that everyone will read *The Golden Thread* because it is a magnificent piece of work that is spiritual and humanly authentic. In truth, that is the highest praise that can be given to a book on spiritual insights.

I also want people to read this book in order to grab hold of Pat's golden thread, to be a part of her brilliant soul, her ethereal grace, and her boundless love. I couldn't bear to say farewell to my beloved friend of so many years but my grief is made easier by her telling us it was her time to go. How privileged we all were to know and to love Pat Pilkington and her beloved Christopher.

Watch over us from the other side until we meet again, darling friend …

Caroline Myss
Oak Park, Illinois, USA

The Golden Thread

Pat Pilkington

Chapter 1
Where do we come from?

"Ever since the dawn of civilisation people have craved an understanding of the underlying order of the world... why it is as it is and why it exists at all." Professor Stephen Hawking, physicist, cosmologist and author of *A Brief History of Time*[1], was speaking at the opening of the London 2012 Paralympic Games. And with a choreographed Big Bang began the brightest, busiest lecture he can ever have conducted.

Over 62,000 people assembled in the Olympic arena, the Queen and royal family, dignitaries and politicians all leaned forward to attend to what was being said. "Look up at the stars," Professor Hawking continued, as a ballet of 62 golden wheelchairs flew high across the stadium and a circle of disabled acrobats stood atop ten foot bendy poles, swaying to the music. All were celebrating the human spirit and the possibilities that lie within us. Professor Hawking, from his wheelchair and hardly able to move a muscle, repeated, "Look up at the stars". Millions watched at home and joined in the sense of wonder: what a world to live in and what a human spirit to celebrate.

Months earlier the same questions were being aired on television by Professor Brian Cox, who asked, "Why are we here? Where do we come from?" He was standing with stars, galaxies and infinite space spread before him in his series *Wonders of the Universe*. Unfolding the amazing cosmic story of the birth and death of stars, he began to say that nothing in the universe is ever lost. New stars are born out of the death of old stars. All is energy, and energy converts, reforms and begins anew. In a bleak, deserted mountainous place in South America, Professor Cox picked up a section of a meteor and, holding it close to the camera, he told his audience to examine some little flecks, dots of coloured matter. "These," he said, "are amino acids, the building blocks of the human body. This," he waved the section in his hand: "this came from the heart of a dying star and it became you and me. We come from the stars." There was awe and triumph in his voice. He was near to tears.

So one answer to the question "where do we come from?" is this: we are energy reformed and we come from the stars. And when we die, as Professor Cox said, we go back into the elements from which we came and we circle and cycle round again.

Professor Stephen Hawking speaks of the triumph of the human spirit and tells us to look up at the stars; Professor Cox says we come from the stars. Science is leading the way.

Why we are here is a more difficult question and one that has puzzled people from the beginning of human consciousness. Having no answer, the only recourse then as now is to look around at the wonders of the world and tell ourselves stories.

In childhood there are few boundaries between what we know is true and what we want to believe is true, and life is shot through with magic. I remember that as a young girl I was aware of another world. It was very close, and sometimes I could almost see into it. There were fairies in the flowers and water sprites dancing on the lake. The descending sun glowed with the magic of this other world and I glowed too. It was familiar and precious and made me feel connected and safe. But when I spoke of it, I was told that I was talking nonsense. It was extremely confusing to know what the 'real' world was. It all seemed real to me.

I remember, too, a sense that I stretched out far beyond my body. Indeed, I had a sense that my body was made of separate parts, distant from each other. I can still recall, eighty years on, the moment when I realised as a very young girl that my body parts were all connected after all. This clear memory of being connected, one piece and whole is vivid and remains with me. I had thought I was lots of little bits, and now I found I was connected!

I look back and think I have gone full circle. As a very small child I knew I was part of everything. I did not feel stuck in one place and solid.

Yet as we grow up we are told we have to deal with the world as it is and live with the fact that we just don't know the answers to our questions. We may try to develop our own belief system, but any kind of faith and belief takes a battering in our modern world where scepticism is highly developed. If you list all the things that you think are true you can guess that someone will give you factual reasons why you are wrong.

As a child I heard with growing incredulity the story of the faith I grew up in: Christianity. The descriptions of Jesus chimed with a remembered familiarity. But the insistence on absolute belief, and the condemnation of non-belief, struck a terribly discordant note. With many others I asked the question "If God is love, how can he condemn his children? I wouldn't do that to a child of mine, and I am not God." No satisfactory answer came, and the fear that underlay this teaching began to eat away the natural inner sense of well-being that had been my familiar state.

As we struggle to understand something undefined, something other worldly, religions have lost no time in creating their own stories to convince us that they hold the key to the universe and that following their rules will bring happiness, contentment and fulfilment. These stories shaped themselves around the things we question most deeply – the mysteries of life and death and our purpose. Religious traditions put in place scriptures and stories as explanations and signposts designed to steer us on a prescribed path. And, as the leaders of religions sought to control the behaviour of a potentially unruly populace, the penalties for straying from the path and for seeking our own truths and ways of being were bound to be harsh in this world and eternal punishment in the next. As a child, I found that my own experience of connection, mystery and magic was in stark contrast to the stories that I was asked to accept from the Christian tradition in which I grew up.

But what if we can continue to make the mysterious other world whisper in our ears as we mature and we journey through the years from birth to death? What if we accept that at a deep and intuitive level we do indeed know something that makes a world of difference?

I believe that inside each of us is a deep part of our being that goes beyond mind and body, that is infused with magic, that gives us a sense of connection and confidence and graces us with an ageless wisdom and perception. This is our inner spirit and it is what I call the Golden Thread. It is something extraordinary that connects and binds us to each other across the generations and to our universe. It is within the wisdom and inspiration that runs through scripture of all faiths if you search for it. 'Golden' because it is shot through with the golden light of divinity; 'Thread' because it joins us together. When we start to become aware of what is threading through our lives, we can see the joined-up pattern of grace and design. The more we look for it, the more we see.

Just as the energy source that brought into being the physical world and all living things is shot through with creative divine power, so are we.

Chapter 2
The Early Years

My childhood was full of acting, dancing and performing, where dressing up and pretending were encouraged. I wanted to be an actress when I grew up and I learned reams of poetry by heart, parts of Shakespeare's plays, and monologues that I hoped might be required at a party. I always had my piece ready for any request that should come.

However, in 1939, into this wonderful childhood came darkness as we were plunged into war with Hitler's Germany. We were evacuated from our family home in Mill Hill, North London, as soon as the war started and some light in me went out. Eileen, my wonderful older sister, did her best to guide and console me, but overwhelming homesickness took its toll and overcame my naturally outgoing nature. Life became serious. We were bombarded with endless warnings about the need to carry a gas mask at all times. Tears and grumbling were met with the retort, "Don't make a fuss. Don't you know there's a war on?" We knew it indeed and nine miserable months of evacuation dragged by until, in May 1940, my father took a house in Hyde Heath in Buckinghamshire and moved us all to be a family again. Eileen and I were reunited with our two little brothers, our parents and grandparents. We were ecstatic.

It was just in time because the 'phoney war' had ended and the terrifying bombing raids had begun. Even in the country we had our share, with nearby bombs bringing down our ceilings and breaking our windows. Being at war was very frightening, but children can always find something to amuse. We searched for shrapnel from the bombs and found a good market among the village boys. What a summer that was. It was too difficult to find schools for us with only a few weeks left of the summer term, and we roamed the countryside on bicycles with a freedom seldom known before or since. Dunkirk, the fall of Paris: dreadful things were happening but this was our first experience of real deep countryside and we were intoxicated by the beauty and the unending delight as the season unfolded.

The only dark moment each day was waiting early in the morning for a phone call from my father, who was sleeping in his London office, to tell us he was all right. There had been firebombs on the roof, he told us, but all had been extinguished. I wonder now, looking back, how my mother endured the strain of it all. A wonderfully energetic, attractive woman, she had to cope with a completely new environment, her husband in harm's way and a house full of children, our own family and several other young people, as well as two aged grannies.

Yet, despite the war, I was still full of my dreams of a theatrical career. When I heard that Sir Henry Wood, famous for the Promenade Concerts, was temporarily residing in a nearby mansion I climbed high into the cherry tree and sang at the top of my voice, hoping he would hear and 'discover' me! News soon came that he had moved back to London. The war was still on and I was going nowhere.

Schools were found for us at the start of the autumn term and after so much freedom it was a shock. With the Battle of Britain going on in the skies above us, we kept a wary eye out for danger as we cycled several miles to school and back. The advice was to lie down in a roadside ditch at the sight of enemy aircraft, but luckily we never had to do it. We were becoming used to the idea of living with danger.

My great good fortune during these dark days was that at

school I made contact with a marvellous drama teacher who encouraged my acting enthusiasm and, after a few years of minor parts, cast me in leading roles in the school plays. She coached me for an audition to enter the Central School of Speech and Drama in London and helped me to win a place there, which I took up in 1946.

The contrast between my time at drama school and my previous existence could not have been greater and I had the happiest three years of my life, with wonderful colleagues and inspiring teachers. But there were no offers for acting jobs on graduation and I took a post in Worcester teaching drama at the Alice Ottley school. So it was that I was there in the city of Worcester when a year or two later a new young curate called Christopher Pilkington was ordained in the Cathedral, and took up his post at a church across town from where I lived. This was going to change everything, though I did not know it at the time.

Some people talk about the two terrible world wars as the death of God, and certainly religious practice has dwindled constantly over the decades since, but during the war ordinary people had gathered in churches up and down the land in answer to a call to prayer. Something of my childhood psychic sense revived in the years after the war, and I felt a direct connection to God that was very powerful. In Worcester I joined a Baptist church and embarked on a bible study course to prepare to join the teachers in the Sunday school. I also became part of a local Christian group that met occasionally in one of the large Worcester houses, and it was there that I first set eyes on Christopher.

The subject for the evening was 'The Proofs of the Resurrection' and the large and gracious room was filled with young people. Our host, a leading doctor in the city, came in once we were all settled and introduced a tall, handsome young man dressed in dark grey suit and clerical collar. My heart turned over! It was a sort of recognition, although of course I had never seen him before. He had a most beautiful voice and, as a voice expert, this made me even more attentive. I was completely captivated and often declared later that I fell in love as soon as he opened his mouth.

What was so strange was that this young curate was taking his talk entirely from a book that I had just read. His headings were the chapter titles; his arguments followed the book exactly. Here was no original work on his part; the credit entirely belonged to the author of the book. Questions followed the talk and quite a lively discussion ensued, in which I took part. When it was clear that the evening was drawing to a close, I guilelessly put the question: "Have you read *Who Moved the Stone?* by Morison[2]?" Christopher paused for just a moment and stuttered out the word "yes", before collapsing with laughter. He knew he had been found out and later, as we passed around the cups of coffee, he came over to talk to me. As we all gathered our coats to leave, he offered me a lift home. "No thank you," I said, "I have my bike."

What was it that made me so honest? How could I not have left my bike to collect the next day, and gone with him? At least he might have got my name and address. But as it was I peddled like a mad thing up the hill to my flat, cursing my foolishness and bewailing the lost opportunity. I was completely captivated and could do nothing about it.

When 1952 moved into 1953, Worcester was planning great things for the new young Queen's coronation. One of the many events was a great production of the mediaeval mystery play 'Everyman' in the Cathedral, and I was very involved, both as an actor and in the production. The director contacted me one day and said she was looking for a well-proportioned young man to play the part of Beauty. She wanted a good voice and figure, and reckoned the rest could be induced by costume and make up. "I know exactly the person," I responded eagerly. "He is the new curate at St John's and he is very good looking."

I heard nothing for a couple of weeks and was eating my heart out, wondering if Christopher would be there at the next rehearsal. I was bathed in disappointment when the day arrived and a quick scan of the Cathedral chapter house revealed no Christopher. I was almost beyond speaking my part with disappointment, but at the end of the rehearsal the director said, "Thank you for telling me about the curate. He couldn't come tonight because he had a confirmation class, but he will be here on Thursday." I was speechless with pleasure and relief and counted the hours and the moments.

So it was that we acted in the same play and got to know each other over the coming weeks. My quaint, old-fashioned headmistress heard rumours that I was walking out with the curate of St John's and she summoned me to her study. Being called to such meetings was always a terrifying experience and I knocked at her door wondering what awaited me. I was tremendously surprised by the roundabout way she approached the subject but finally got the concealed message: Christopher and I were both notable figures in the city of Worcester; he a priest and I a teacher at the prestigious school. Would I please be sure that we behaved at all times with decorum and dignity...? She smiled and added that she was sure I would understand. What I did understand was that we had to meet far enough away from the old lady's spies. Christopher was angry at such interference, but we agreed to skip over the hills to beautiful Malvern for our rendezvous in future.

· · · · · · ·

We were married in August 1954. My father, who had never understood my penchant for churchgoing, thought it apposite I was marrying Christopher - only a vicar would do, he declared! Father was the soul of integrity and charity and was brought up by a pious and deeply religious mother, yet the horrors he had lived through in the trenches of the First War had killed any religious belief. What he considered was slight religious oddity in both bride and groom was made up for by learning that Christopher was part of a wealthy Lancashire family who had made money in the glassmaking business. Why hadn't I mentioned it, he asked. He was absolutely confused when I said that I simply hadn't known about it. He couldn't believe he had raised such a simpleton!

After a brief honeymoon I settled happily into the curate's flat and a new life of joy and love that was beyond my wildest dreams. In less than a year Christopher was offered a parish of his own called St Mark in the Cherry Orchard, and we moved into our first house on the other side of Worcester. Our real life together had begun.

Before we moved to the new parish, however, only months after hosting our wedding so graciously, my father died from a cerebral haemorrhage. He was only sixty two. The strange thing was that his identical twin brother had also died just four days earlier. They had both survived the First World War and now it looked as if their shared life-energy had run out at almost identical moments. My family were deeply grief-stricken, and so was I. My church taught that only committed Christians would progress in the afterlife, and the thought that tormented me was that I had seen my beloved father for the last time. "Tell me I will see him again," I sobbed in Christopher's arms and, though he tried to comfort me, it was as though he were not entirely certain. The pain went on for many weeks and only ended when I met Tim Tiley, the vicar of a neighbouring parish.

The Reverend Tim Tiley was a talented and gifted healer, but Christopher didn't know this when he invited him to preach at Harvest Festival Evensong in our new church. I scurried home at the end of the service to get the supper ready and, in due course, the two men came back to the vicarage to eat. Tim was some years older than us and was charming and easy to talk to. After all the usual polite conversation that graced the start of our meal, Tim began to talk to us about healing - what the Church referred to as 'laying on of hands'.

A healer is seen as a channel for positive energy that can help people to heal themselves. Healers usually have robust inner lives from regular spiritual practice of one sort or another that allows them to be in close contact with the source of healing energy. Healing appears to work on all levels: spiritual, mental, emotional and physical.

Tim told us the extraordinary story of how healing came into his life. When he was a boy, he had 'died' of double pneumonia. In the 1950s almost no-one spoke about near-death experience and I remember vividly my incredulity as he told his story. He said that he lifted out of his body and hovered over it, delighted to be free and out of pain. He had no sense of fear, or of how strange it was that there now existed two of him. He felt no interest in the body on the bed, but happily and freely moved towards a light that seemed to draw him to the corner of the room. The light opened into a corridor of light, along which he travelled into what he called 'the other world'.

There he was greeted by a host of friends who eagerly escorted him on a tour of the most beautiful place one could ever imagine. Tim never tired of describing the glorious landscapes, the rivers and waterfalls, the flowers, trees and birds. He always ran out of words because it was beyond description. Everything was suffused with glowing light. "Did you see God?" we asked. "God <u>was</u> the light," he answered. Full of questions, young Tim was puzzling in his mind, "Who can come here?" and immediately an answer came loud and clear in his consciousness. "Everyone comes here. You are all welcomed home by Love. You take your journey to earth for Love's sake, and Love welcomes you home." "Everyone?" I exclaimed. "Surely not - what about Hitler?" Tim gently said, "Even Hitler will get there in the end."

A 'being of light', who the young Tim took to be the Lord, asked him if he would be willing to return to earth to work for God. Tim said, "All I wanted was to stay in that marvellous place, but you don't say no when someone like that asks you!" And the next thing he knew was that he was back in his body, with his life to live ahead of him. But he had not come back empty-handed. He had a marvellous gift of healing, and he also retained the ability to ask a question in his mind and receive a direct answer from a heavenly guide. No wonder he was so wonderful to be with, and no wonder his teaching was so vivid, exciting and compassionate. Tim turned on all the lights of Heaven for us and after meeting him everything sparkled with a new glory.

It was from Tim that Christopher and I began to understand that a great deal of the Christian theology and dogma that we had learned since childhood was man-made. With Tim's help we recovered the essence of connection that we had both known in our infant days but that we struggled to find in our church life. God, Tim said, was Light and Love. It was not helpful to think in human terms of a God-person being out there … like fish in the sea, he said, we swim in an ocean of God energy. If you ask a fish what it thinks of the ocean, it would say, "What ocean? We are what we are." So with us: we are so familiar with the energy and vibrations around us that we take them for granted. Only when we turn our heads a little, feeling the presence, do we begin to sense the connection.

Could it be true that the stories of scripture that we have learned over the years were needed because the mind cannot comprehend something so abstract as energy and vibration? To form a commitment to a higher power you have to have a relationship with it and it has to engage the heart. Connection with the Divine need not come from creeds and dogmas but from the raising of our energetic vibration, by tuning in to the sea of love that flows all around us and within us. If we do this we strengthen our inner spirit and find that the golden light of divinity shines in our lives. It is that relationship, the relationship of the Golden Thread, that works; the rest is the 'story' that has grown around our faith.

Theologians tell us that Jesus lived and taught and died in Palestine, and that the Christian Church developed after his resurrection. But it is also a fact that stories have an essential and integral truth in and of themselves, whether they are real in a concrete sense, or true metaphorically. We are living our lives on many levels and we intuitively understand the different worlds we inhabit: the world of fact and the world of fantasy. We don't have to explain them all the time. We live by factual, scientific truth when that is important to us, and we live at another, mystical level when our hearts open in rapture, when we are connected.

We were so captivated to sit and talk to Tim, someone who had visited the 'other world', in such a relaxed and easy way. Our questions followed one after the other. And Tim could answer each one. We had never heard anything like this in all of our lives. Out came my real grief: would I see my father again? "Of course," Tim answered. How could it be otherwise? None of the words that actually came from the mouth of Jesus said anything about such separation. Tim said that the words of judgement that we now read in the New Testament were added later. The early leaders of the Church gathered the sayings of Jesus after the resurrection and edited them into volumes in the fourth century. Much that was already written was discarded and Church teaching was added to try to make it clear to the ever-growing body of followers what they should believe and how they should live. Dogma and doctrine were woven into the original story, which started out as a simple story of love.

All this was absolutely new to me. I had never questioned or doubted the origin of what I had been taught as a child or what I learned as an adult when I studied the Bible as part of my daily practice. I had been assured that it was the word of God and simply never questioned it. But here was Tim, so clearly sincere and well informed, and a clergyman to boot, turning a lot of my beliefs upside down. I was enchanted but not convinced. Christopher, on the other hand, had spent five years at Cambridge studying theology and preparing for ordination and knew and understood more of what we were being told. He had seen the many anomalies and contradictions that face any scholar of early Christianity. He also had a sense of the growing power of the early Church authorities; they had something in the nature of a rushing wind or roaring fire to deal with. So great was the enthusiasm among newly converted believers that it could all run out of control - a strong hand was needed and, of course, that is what prevailed. Dogma and doctrine were taught and enforced in order to maintain control as Christianity spread.

We were still sitting at the supper table hours later that Sunday night. We had been captivated by this new way of seeing life and death and the evening had flown by. Tim's wife Mystica phoned anxiously at 1am asking if all was well. Luckily she was very forgiving and thus began a friendship that endured for the next thirty years. They generously lent us books, introduced us to the ministry of healing and guided our uncertain steps until at last we were able to accept a whole new way of seeing this world and the next.

Christopher always said that healing was the greatest help to his work in the parish. Whatever the problem, there was always something that could be done to help. We spent long hours talking about it and began to dream that one day, far in the future, we would have a healing sanctuary. In my mind's eye I saw a gracious Georgian house, and a beautiful garden with a wonderful cedar tree.

In the event it took twenty years to materialise exactly as I had seen it!

They were twenty busy years. Three children came to bless and complete our lives. We made another move, this time close to Birmingham, to a large parish called St John's, Bromsgrove where our third child John was born.

After being in a small and manageable parish in Worcester, moving to Bromsgrove was a shock! The house was enormous, with a front stairs and back stairs, corridors of flagstones downstairs and seven bedrooms upstairs. Every church meeting (and there were lots of them) took place in the vicarage because there was no parish hall. The garden was the size of a park and every parish event took place in it, so Christopher and I were surrounded by people all day. A bereaved and aged aunt with cancer also moved in with us and lived her last year as part of our family. I saw the carefree young man I had married age in front of my eyes. There seemed no end to the work when God is your boss.

All through this time, however, Tim was there to help. He regularly came to give my aunt healing. Breast cancer progressed into the bone and inevitably there was pain but it was held at bay. We saw the power of healing in action. At the time I didn't realise what an amazing thing this was, but looking back it is clear that something extraordinary was taking place. I was able to take my aunt in the car to a nearby churchyard full of snowdrops in flower at the end of February. She gazed and gazed at the wonderful sight. We slowly walked up the path and into the church, to sit in a pew and read the service of Evensong:

> *Lord, now lettest thou thy servant depart in peace,*
> *according to thy word;*
> *For mine eyes have seen thy salvation.*

My aunt died two days later.

• • • • • • •

In the midst of life, we are in death. And what do we do? We cope with it, and we take a deep breath and get on with life, but we ponder on how much we need tradition and ritual to get us through. There is an endless questing to find answers to the meaning of life. We are faced with such a mystery and so much difficulty on the path from birth to death that we need some shared belief to make sense of it and bring us together. Although at the time I did not articulate the thought, it began to form as a distant concept: we need a story that is told and retold from generation to generation, whether it has a background in actual truth or is a satisfying and accepted legend. Truth is less important than the message it tells. The story has to speak to our hearts as we go through the valley of the shadow of death. We need some form of spirituality to uphold our spirits and lighten our load. I had begun to take my first faltering steps in the exploration of what that spirituality might be, and it was not easily found in the conventional Church in which we were working.

Chapter 3
A Developing Spirituality, and a New Healing Centre

A round the time of our move to Bromsgrove came the news that the early Christian Gnostic Gospels, discovered buried in the sand in Egypt in 1945, were being partially published and were available to purchase. Christopher had little time for study in those days with the mountain of work that he faced daily, but this was an especial interest and he made time for it.

The term Gnosis comes from the Greek for 'knowledge', by which is meant 'inner knowing'. Ultimately it means knowledge of who we really are, where we come from, how we got here and how we can return. Gnostics taught that the world is a place of imprisonment where sparks of the Divine are trapped in human bodies. Inner knowledge, or gnosis, is needed to make the return. When this knowledge is received, they said, it is like a sleeper awakening, or a drunken man becoming sober, as the 'good news' frees the soul to make its return back home. Gnostic texts are full of heartfelt gratitude to God for the unexpected salvation (gnosis) that has been received.

This was deemed to be heresy by the emerging Christian Church and orders went out to destroy all Gnostic texts; no doubt this was why the Gnostic gospels were buried in jars and dug deep into the sand in the third or fourth century. It would be seventeen hundred years before they were accidentally dug up and rediscovered. At the time however, starting with St Paul, the early Church was beginning to teach that salvation came through belief in the death and resurrection of Jesus Christ. It was a matter of salvation by one's faith in God rather than inner knowing. The Gnostics taught that we are a spark and a hologram of the Divine, containing the same properties as the Divine, albeit on a minuscule scale. It is not a matter of substance; it is a matter of degree. If we see the Divine as the source of creation, then it follows that we holographic sparks are creators too.

If you visit any large bookshop you will see lined up on the shelves all sorts of books such as *The Law of Attraction, The Power of Intention, The Secret, Bring out the Magic in Your Mind, Jung and Synchronicity*, and so forth. All these send out the message that we have an enormous power to create and shape the world around us. You may think we haven't made a very good job of it but, even if there is a grain of truth in between the covers, then we must give some attention to the way we can influence the world around us. How we can do this is a whole other story, but for now the starting point is to look for the answer to the eternal questions: who am I, where did I come from, how did I get here, where am I going, and to what purpose?

A Gnostic may be refreshingly clear on these questions and answer: "I am a spark of the Divine, I incarnate from the other world, I am going to live a fully conscious, joyous and intentional life, the purpose is to love and be loved; to enlarge my experience, develop soul strength, and bring light to all around me. Finally I will take this great work back to the other world, where I am known and loved, understood and eagerly awaited." The starting point is to be open to the thought that the soul is immortal, a part of the Divine, existing before and after this physical adventure.

Certainly those answers present a startlingly uncomplicated approach: we are shot through with divine power and can achieve transcendence and salvation for ourselves. It is like a key within each of us that can be turned. This personal transcendence is born of love and inner knowing and is far removed from fear-inducing rigid religious dogma. Is that why the emerging Christian Church wanted to bury the Gnostic Gospels?

• • • • • • •

I have a dear neighbour, a retired headmistress, who once spent some time in hospital. She had been undergoing tests and at night was able only to doze fitfully in the noisy ward. She came to in the early hours to see her brother standing at the foot of her bed. Although she knew this to be unusual, she was not at all alarmed. She couldn't exactly recall what he said, but remembered vividly that he was assuring her that everything was all right. The next day she was told that he had died the night before. As she told me this story, she said that it made perfect sense to her, and that knowing he was all right made all the difference. "I have not wept for him," she said.

"I shall miss him a great deal, but I know he is alive and that he will keep in touch. Indeed," she said, "He has come several times since. He always stands at the foot of my bed and tells me that all is well. Since that first visit I have been told that I have pancreatic cancer. I think now when he comes, he is reassuring me that I am going to be all right. It is very comforting."

I have heard similar stories over and over again. People often say that they haven't told anyone before, for fear of being thought crazy. Hearing me talk about the next world has somehow given them permission to speak at last.

More and more I feel certain that knowledge of the next world is vital to finding a satisfactory way to live in this one. As with any journey, it is vital to know where you are coming from, and where you are going. Once we know that there is a purpose and a destination to the journey of life, then we can settle down to make the very best of our time here. It is a waste of a precious lifetime not to enjoy our wonderful world and the joys of living and loving. Even pitting our strength against difficulties can feel physically and mentally rewarding; it is empowering to find out how strong we are. How can we know we are courageous if we have no dragons to fight? I often hear cancer patients saying that they cannot go through more treatment, or endure more uncertainty then later, when it is all behind them, they find they were stronger than they thought. It is always reassuring.

Courage is a soul strength, so is patience and endurance and we seem to find circumstances that allow us to practise these virtues. Think about it: how do I know that I have a loving and forgiving nature unless I am challenged to work at a deep soul level in order to be able to forgive and love? Does knowing how this works make it easier? The answer is "no", but it does at least give a possible reason for what a situation is doing in my life.

Undoing the constricting templates of our existing life and opening to a larger frame of growth and development brings tension and sometimes tears but, once we understand the process of this oft-repeated exercise, we can allow it to happen with more grace and ease. We are reaching deep into our true nature and allowing more of our essence to show through. We observe this happening to people around us and say that they are becoming more mature and resourceful: re-Source-full. They, and we, are plugged into the Divine Source and taking more from it.

> Recognise what is before your eyes,
> And what is hidden will be revealed to you.[3]

• • • • • • •

In Christopher's family it was a tradition that children went to good public schools for their secondary education. Our two sons and daughter were still tiny but names had to be registered in good time, so on some of our very rare expeditions we went to look over a number of schools in the South West. I enjoyed these outings very much indeed and was interested to be entertained by headmasters and shown around grand and impressive buildings.

Christopher and his brothers had all been to Clifton College in Bristol, so that was on our list. We found it extremely impressive and just close by was a marvellous school for our daughter. We decided to register them and began filling in forms. There was one thing, however, that I could not face. I did not want our children to become boarders so I begged Christopher to allow us to enter the children as day pupils. "How are you planning to get them here every morning early when we live a hundred miles away?" he asked, raising his eyebrows. I replied that perhaps we could rent a flat for weekdays, and come home at weekends. Although it was not exactly a practical idea, we nevertheless put them down to be day pupils.

Some time later a letter came out of the blue to our vicarage in Bromsgrove, offering Christopher the job of Rector of the City Parish of St Stephen's in the centre of Bristol! I can remember standing in the kitchen with the letter in my hands, astonished and unbelieving. How could such a thing be happening? What extraordinary power was at work that answered our need in such an amazing way? Who delivered the message that we wanted our children to go to school in Bristol? What strange sort of world did we live in that could accommodate our heartfelt wishes so neatly? We moved to Bristol in 1968 but it was years before we began to understand the power of thought and intention that can bring about such synchronous events.

Dr Wayne Dyer, in his book *The Power of Intention*[4], says the energy that surrounds us can be tuned into so that people can become what he calls 'connectors' who trust an invisible source to provide what they need. He quotes Carlos Castaneda in his opening chapter:

> *In the universe there is an immeasurable, indivisible*
> *force which shamans call intent and absolutely*
> *everything that exists in the entire cosmos is attached*
> *to intent by a connecting link.*

Could this be the Golden Thread of my imagining? Could it be an invisible field of energy that we can tune in to, not by striving or force of will, but by aligning with it and experiencing it? Where is this field? "There's no place that it's not," says Dr Dyer. "If you cut open an acorn you won't see a giant oak tree, but you know it's there. Every aspect of nature, without exception, has intention built into it. At our source we are formless vibrating energy of infinite potential. Activating intention means rejoining your Source and becoming a modern day sorcerer." Once again, it seems that a single thought can change the world. Certainly we had somehow found a way to do this very thing, without even trying, and we were to go on pulling rabbits out of hats again and again in the years to come.

With your thoughts you make the world, as Buddha said[5], and the premise is that thought affects reality; that reality is not fixed but fluid and open to influence. Elite sportsmen and women have known this for a long time, as have healers and other metaphysical practitioners. This is the basis of their work. How do they do it? Wayne Dyer says, "Expand your reality to the point where you pursue what you love doing and excel at it. Involve yourself in the high-energy levels of trust, optimism, appreciation, reverence, joy and love; trust your insights, and meditate."

Without knowing what we were doing, clearly we were fulfilling some of those instructions because very soon after Christopher started as Rector of St Stephen's, people began to come to him, telling him that they were healers. They had heard he was starting a healing ministry. Well, it was true but he hadn't said a word to anyone about it. He was too busy getting to know his new area of work. The other strange thing that had happened was that our teacher and friend, Reverend Tim Tiley, had been offered a living about twenty miles north of Bristol so he was also on the move, and would still be a near neighbour.

There was a great deal of sadness in the Bromsgrove parish as we left, and we were not prepared for it. Eight years of developing his ministry skills had made Christopher a very popular vicar and people were truly upset that he was going. Tears were flowing when he held his final service and we were showered with gifts as tokens of appreciation.

A wonderful preacher, Christopher had taught and encouraged people in the way Tim had shown him. He made Jesus so real to the people, and had somehow joined this world and the next world in such a way that death was seen as a navigable horizon. We felt terribly sad to be leaving them all, although we sincerely wanted to go to Bristol. Our young children were leaving the only home they knew and all their friends and it took all of us quite a long time to settle into our new life. The children had to go to new schools and we faced a new parish. It felt very hard work for us all, especially Christopher, but eventually we settled into our new home and began to get our bearings.

The rectory in Bristol had eight bedrooms and we were expected to do quite a lot of entertaining. We were also invited to endless civic occasions and grand functions that required a new wardrobe! We missed the prayer ministry and the healing groups that had become part of our Bromsgrove life, and this all felt a bit more superficial. So when yet another healer turned up saying that she had heard about a new healing ministry, Christopher thought he might as well get started. To begin with we opened a Natural Health Support Group in the church hall and from that the healing gradually developed.

I also auditioned for BBC Radio Bristol that had recently begun broadcasting and was taken on as a freelance reporter. My first boss was Kate Adie and I had ten wonderful years making radio documentaries - years full of interest and creativity. Now that we had settled, we could see that Bristol was a really marvellous place to be.

Amongst our new contacts were three very experienced healers and Christopher began to let it be known that the City Parish of St Stephen's was open for healing each week at certain times. It was extraordinary how people came. We only had the church as a venue and it was open of course for visitors. The constant stream of tourists, guided round its mediaeval marvels by the verger, made the sort of peace and quiet we wanted almost impossible; as the years passed and the healing ministry grew, Christopher and I began to talk about finding another place. We wondered about renting somewhere suitable, but couldn't imagine where or what sort of place.

Christopher's father died in 1975 and, as if on cue, during the time we were considering finding new premises came the news that we had inherited a legacy under the terms of his will. We felt blessed and were spurred on into looking at properties that we could buy to set up a proper healing centre. Tim Tiley was still closely involved and was very keen on the idea and helped us choose a really beautiful house in Downfield Road near the Downs in leafy Clifton. It was far too big for what we needed and we turned two floors into flats, just using the ground floor for the healing work. It was a very good time to buy, the mid 70s, just before the big property boom. In the long run every inch of this house would be used for the work of the Bristol Cancer Help Centre. How much, I wonder looking back, were we bringing the future into being? As with many things in our lives, we seemed to be in the right place at the right time.

With a property for our healing centre secured, it made us think that we also ought to invest in a property for ourselves. We lived in a rectory that, of course, didn't belong to us and in the event of accident or death we would have to find somewhere else to live. We talked to Tim and his wife Mystica about where and how to find exactly the right place.

Mystica, true to her name, lived a life of prayer and devotion. In answer to my question she said, "You must just ask God to find for you a place perfect for your needs - He knows them. And ask that someone will be as happy to sell to you as you are to buy." She told me to say this prayer with mind and heart fully engaged. I thought it sounded pretty simple and nearly forgot to do so but, strangely, that evening when I went to our bedroom in the rectory I was attracted by the late sunshine lighting up the view over Clifton and the crowded streets wending their way out to the Somerset countryside. It looked absolutely beautiful. Something triggered the memory of Mystica's words and with a full heart I spoke the words aloud.

Very soon a communication arrived in the post from an estate agent we had consulted in Wells, bearing details of an isolated and semi-derelict eighteenth century gamekeeper's cottage on the Mendip Hills, surrounded by fields and with extensive views. By evening we had viewed the property and had dropped the deposit through the agent's letterbox to secure it for us. When I told Mystica on the phone, all she said was, "Of course! A prayer like that always works."

Our new healing centre in Downfield Road went under the name of The Guy Pilkington Foundation, in memory of Christopher's father, and Tim agreed to teach there. We began to gather an ever-increasing circle of people around us who wanted to train as healers. In those early years the centre attracted about a dozen healers who worked there on a voluntary basis and visitors were offered their services for free. Tim and Christopher led the training but I would also occasionally set up an evening meeting for everyone and invite a natural health practitioner to come and talk about their work. Through this we made wonderful contacts with naturopaths, homoeopaths, chiropractors and osteopaths and we welcomed anyone who wanted to come for alternative therapies and to learn yoga and meditation and receive healing.

One evening my invited guest was Penny Brohn, an acupuncturist and practitioner of Chinese medicine. We didn't know that this was to start something that would take over our lives, but Christopher and I were captivated by Penny's beauty and charisma. Intelligent, charming and fascinating, we were delighted when she began to come to Tim's evenings regularly. With her husband David, and three young children, Penny became part of our ever-widening circle. It was clear that the healing ministry was bringing towards us people who wanted to deepen their spiritual practice and their inner lives, and both Christopher and Tim had a wonderful way of helping people to do just that. They brought a clarity that made it all so attractive.

Chapter 4
Tuning into Love

Spirituality, of course, does not arrive without effort. Religions have all demonstrated a requirement for constant attention: people are instructed to go to church, temple or mosque regularly, and at appointed times. We are taught to meditate and pray; we are encouraged to study and join in fellowship. We begin to understand that the soul needs an intense, full-bodied spiritual life as much as the body needs food. Soul work is alchemy, pilgrimage and adventure.

Caroline Myss, in *Entering the Castle*[6], says that today "we are mystics without monasteries". In days gone by, people with a spiritual quest would enter an Order and have a daily programme carved out for them in the routine of the religious life. Worship, prayer, study and household tasks followed each other, sweetened by a little recreation. Anyone having a physical or spiritual temper tantrum, Caroline says, was sent to the kitchen to peel potatoes! It wouldn't suit us now; we are far too individualistic. But today's budding mystics have to find this rhythm of devotion within the noise and bustle of modern daily life. "When should I pray or meditate?" we ask. "I am too rushed in the morning and too tired at night. I have too much to do in my free time to attend a place of worship: the children have cricket, tennis, music practice ... there just isn't a moment." Perhaps the monastery is beginning to look a bit more attractive! Surrounded as we are by noise and traffic, television, mobile phones and endless activity, our over-burdened systems are crying out for peace and quiet. So people go fishing, they walk the dog, they run, they hike in the country, they garden and they go to concerts. Intuitively something in us is searching for relief and a way of living a spiritual reality in the present. Caroline Myss writes:

> "How will you come for me, Lord? How will I know you? How will I recognise you?

> "I know you will come for me. You will slip into my being, perhaps in the middle of the night while I sleep.

> "Maybe you will come for me when I am not looking for you, when I am distracted, staring into an oncoming storm, fearing my immortality."

> And God replies:

> "You are my creation. I know you. I know your every thought, your every action, your every breath. You are one with me."

· · · · · · ·

We all found the spiritual life in Tim's company as rewarding and exciting as it had ever been. The Gnostics spoke of being truly awake, and this was what it felt like. Life before, by comparison, was an out-of-focus picture. Now everything was in sharp relief and it was so much easier. It was like tuning in to a symphonic note ringing out in the cosmos and having ears trained to the full range of its rapture. There is in fact a great deal of sound around us that we simply do not hear. I have a colony of bats in my roof, but I can't hear the sounds they make. When an expert came with a little machine that lowered the pitch, then I could hear their chatter. Might it be so with eternal cosmic sound – with a little help we can all hear it?

Each human energy state has what could be called its note, its own vibration: low for deep depressive states, and high for joy, optimism, love and spiritual union. In between ranges an ascending and descending scale denoting the full range of emotional states of vibration. Such a sound system has an echo in human scale attachments and relationships. In infancy some things clearly raise the spirits and the vibration of the child. Pleasure at the breast, in the mother's arms; play, contentment and joy clearly enable the child to rise up the emotional scale. Such bliss quickens the vibration and raises the baby's emotional and physical wellbeing. The happy child affects the vibrational field around it, and draws a response, as like calls to like. So we are like giant tuning forks, playing off each other, and raising or lowering the field of vibration around us.

When something we experience is reliably found to 'hit the spot' and induce the bliss response, we return to it many times for another shot of 'bliss brain chemicals'. Touching, loving, dancing, running, music, drama, poetry, nature and beauty all raise the emotional vibration and increase the feel-good endorphins. As we understand it, the highest and purest vibration is Divinity itself. We instinctively speak of things being heavenly, and rapture is 'seventh heaven'. Spiritual traditions have always spoken of another world: a place of beauty and peace, which souls may enter after death. Such a world, they tell us, is not separate, but near and fully engaged with us. Where a loving relationship exists, it echoes back our heightened vibration and many who have lost a loved one feel closeness still. Psychics and mystics teach themselves to become entrained to that higher vibration and can maintain a reliable and reproducible contact.

For the rest of us, over a lifetime we usually slowly rise in the scale of awareness, whether we believe in such things or not. We fall in love, we give birth, and we become less selfish and self-absorbed. We open to the needs of others and often with pain and sorrow we learn of the fragility of life. We begin to look for things that do not fade, and this sometimes leads to adopting beliefs and practices that make us feel better and less vulnerable. So communities gather for worship and prayer, others take to the hills to commune with nature, some literally vibrate to pop music or join a quiet throng in a concert hall. All have in common the ability to move from low states of being to the high vibration of joy, bliss and communion.

So we may consider that what we think of as 'heaven' is actually a vibration, a high one. Most of the time we do not feel in contact with such a high state of being but we generally move in and out according to how we are feeling. It could be that when we are able to raise our vibration high enough we touch Divinity. I touch and experience a high vibration of bliss and joy when I pray, when I hold my baby, when I walk in my garden, when I make love, and when I listen to Mozart. The experience is absolutely real and, to me as a Christian, it is evidence of God within me. It shows itself in the vibrancy of my being; it can be measured and it is quantifiable. I know of nothing that is more real that this. Is God real? Yes. He is real to me.

If we are experiencing misery, pain and dejection, we can say we are going through hell. If feeling in a blissful or 'heavenly' state is a state of high energy or vibration, then in contrast 'hell' or depression can be said to be a low state of energy or vibration. If we could learn to move from a low state to a higher state, what a difference it could make to our lives.

Explaining how vibration can be raised is helpful, because people can then set out on a positive way of learning how to do it themselves. It is a journey not a race and no penalties exist for how long it takes. We can go above or beyond what is expected or normal and access a state above mere humanness. We can enter into the area of our 'Divine Spark', linked together by the Golden Thread.

This may be a long way from the things that you believe or have been taught in the past. It took me a long time to dare to look at my 'received wisdom' in a new light - I feared losing all my brownie points! It was childish, I know, but I really felt that someone was counting. I was truly afraid to let go. Then one day the words of Jesus from St John's Gospel jumped out at me:

You will know the Truth and the Truth will set you free.[7]

And I thought to myself, if I am afraid, then I am not free, so this cannot be the truth. Did I rise up, free at last? I wish I could say that I did, but in truth it was a long, slow process. I realised that the older I was getting, the lighter I was beginning to feel. I was discarding many things that had weighed me down, especially my learned religious dogma of an ancient pattern of a world, with heaven up in the sky, earth in the middle and hell below.

It became easier to abandon this view in the light of modern knowledge. We now know that a great deal of what we had been taught in the past was the stuff of legends and stories that pointed to metaphor, not reality. So it became easier to explore further. With no heaven 'up there', where did the old man on the cloud sit to judge the earth and hand out laws and punishments? This too was a myth. So, if He wasn't there, where was He? Did He exist at all?

Many of us are longing to find a home for our spirituality, to awaken, revive and connect with the non-material world. Where can we find that unified field, that divine matrix that contains 'all' and yet is intimately close and intensely personal? Can we stand in the river of life's streaming and choose a new image of what it means to be human?

In the Gnostic Gospel of Thomas there is a reply:

Cleave the wood and you will find me;
Lift a stone and I am there.[8]

Sensing the truth of this, the soul revives in a flash of energy and finds the source of its being: love, divine love and human love. It recovers its purpose in coming to live this lifetime. It has come to give and receive love.

When we come to earth we become entrapped in the physical experience, enjoying human life and rising to its challenges. Then the going gets tough and something within us awakens a longing to be free and to connect again with the spiritual world. We learn from the down times as well as the happy times and slowly make progress.

Over a lifetime much is achieved and we can begin to rise above the chaos of the world and connect to eternity. How do we do this? It takes understanding, focus and practice. It is the same for any expert in their field: athletes train many hours a day, focusing on health, exercise and strength. Musicians often start at an extraordinarily young age, practising many hours a day, their talent becoming their passion. A perfect performance on a track, a field or in a concert hall is the culmination of absolute dedication, discipline and hard work.

The same is true for entrepreneurs and leaders in the field of commerce and business. Ask how many hours Bill Gates put in before he developed Microsoft; think of the years of study and practice that is needed to prepare a surgeon to lift up his scalpel. The same principle applies in the spiritual life: we work to develop higher states of consciousness, insight, grace and peace. We work to bring things that normally apply to the spiritual plane into the earthly environment, through healing energy and raised consciousness. Do we do these things as a challenging duty? I don't think so. We do them because it is our joy and our delight, and because we find that they work.

I am reminded of a story told of Mother Teresa of Calcutta. Someone said that it was a miracle that she and her nuns could do such work. "The miracle," she said, "is not that we do this work, but that we love to do it." It echoes the saying of Jesus – "It is my meat and my drink to do the will of my father and to finish his work."[9]

Joy and delight are high-energy states and the power to change things that they produce, like a good working dynamo, makes further positive emotion. When I was a child in the war we cycled everywhere. The roads were almost empty of traffic, so cycling was a pleasure, as well as the only way to get about. In winter we had to have lights that worked in order to see our way home from school. We had some device fixed to the wheels that made a dynamo work and, as long as we were pedalling, the lights were on. If we stopped, the lights went out. It was not ideal! To have light, we had to keep up the effort. In the same way, to have high and positive energy and joy, we need to keep practising. Practising what? Practising whatever takes you into those delectable high-energy states: gratitude, prayer, praise, stillness, and sensing a heavenly presence in ordinary everyday things.

Caroline Myss refers to something that she calls her 'grace bank account'[10]. You know how you put money regularly into a bank account to keep it topped up for use? In the same way, she says, you can have a 'grace bank account' which you keep topped up with all the things that lift your heart. So when you linger over a rose bush and smell the gorgeous perfume, you think to yourself, this lovely scent is filling up my grace bank account. Indeed, the whole garden on a sunny morning makes its way there. As does the sweet song of a robin, the taste of a fresh apple, the smile from a baby and anything else that delights heart and soul.

In times of leisure and in places of beauty we can feel that we are brimming with grace. It comes in many ways and at different times and allows us to be gracious to the world around us. Love is the great enhancer of grace and they say that 'all the world loves a lover'. Of course it does! The expanded heart of someone in love radiates high voltage energy that sweetens and cheers.

We need to practise ways to get us through the ups and downs of life in the easiest and most graceful way possible. Just look to find something that works. If that is a faith and a religion, then use the symbolism that goes with your belief. If you feel that there is nothing out there, then use the power of your heart and mind, your imagination and your perception to lever yourself into a higher energy state. One day we may have a little machine to test our energy state, like blood pressure gauges. But for now just ask your built-in barometer, "How is this making me feel?" and you may be told how to proceed. If, like my old bicycle light, the energies are dimming, then we know we need to build up our grace bank account. As Guy Brown says in *The Energy of Life*[11]:

> *It may be more important for our overall well-being to track our feelings of energy than to follow our calorie intake or bank accounts.*

Chapter 5
Heavy Burdens

By Autumn 1978, once the summer holidays were over, the programme of healing started once more at our healing centre, together with our evening meetings with Tim. A message came from Penny Brohn telling us of the sudden and unexpected death of her father. He was no great age and she was devastated, together with her family. When we saw her, she was pale and sad. It was her first experience of family loss and the tears came readily. We were so sorry and wondered what we could do to help. I recalled my own terrible sense of loss many years before when my own father died.

The days passed and things were beginning to return to some sort of normality when, exactly eight weeks from her father's death, Penny's mother had a heart attack and died in Penny's arms. Penny's shock and devastation was extreme. Later she told me that the experience was compounded by the fact that as she tried resuscitation and called the ambulance, two angels joined her: one at her mother's feet, one at her head. After a few moments they carefully lifted some essence from the body and departed. In any other situation, such a visitation would have been a cause for wonder but to say that Penny mourned her loss hardly expresses what it meant to her. Her parents were her rock and a solid source of support.

With her sisters, Penny faced the difficult task of clearing and selling the house. It was months of work and intense sadness that were still taking their toll when the year moved into 1979. We all hoped to see some lifting of mood but Penny seemed low-spirited and lacking energy. As the spring turned to summer news filtered through that Penny had found a lump in her left breast. There seemed to be a long time of uncertainty as the year progressed, but finally came the confirmation that it was cancer. She was thirty-six, and it was an unbelievable shock for her and her family, and for all of us who knew and loved her.

Penny was told that she needed a mastectomy and that the operation would take place in a hospital in Bath. A great circle of prayer was formed around her and we waited anxiously for news. It was as if our honeymoon with healing and prayer at the centre in Clifton was at an end. What happened to the joy and the sense of communion when dark clouds were gathering overhead? Someone close to Penny suggested that she got down on her knees and confessed her sins to a god who was punishing her. We were all aghast that such a thought was possible, but it was clear that a lot of the old heavy belief remained hiding in the dark.

Where did we learn that our journey through life was going to be such hard work? Was it from a parent, a teacher, a preacher? Who gave them such authority? It seems to go back a long way. "With the sweat of your brow will you bring forth…", God was supposed to say to our poor old ancestor as he cast him out of paradise. And don't forget the miserable wife: "with sorrow shalt thou bring forth…", condemning poor Eve to hard labour. With our mother's milk we took in the message that we should give ourselves a hard time. It is no wonder that we hardly know how to relax and make things work for us. There is a huge weight of guilt that hangs over our heads from the moment that we are born, if we are to believe some of the stories of judgement and divine punishment from those who have gone before us.

This theme runs through the Old Testament and into the New, and it has shaped western thought for two thousand years. It is deeply ingrained in the way we think about ourselves, even though in modern times most people are unaware of where this burden of guilt comes from. Though few today practise faith or believe in any demonstrable way, nevertheless there is a sense of a lurking, judging power 'out there'. Some even believe the cataclysms that befall our lives come from a punishing God. It is a crude and violent way of looking at life, and I choose not to believe it.

The picture of religion that many of us have inherited is based in a frighteningly violent world, but there is also the possibility of the upward path of transcendence. Jesus taught about a God of Love. It was his gift to the world. Everything that Jesus did and said reinforced this concept of love and transcendence. He spoke of joy and abundant life. He told of the care that the Father has towards us. He adored children and said that they belonged to the kingdom with their trusting natures and joyous optimism. He spoke of forgiveness and eternal life. "Fear not" was constantly on his lips. His was a teaching completely without judgement. How do Jesus' words of love marry with the contrasting teachings of divine retribution and original sin in other parts of the bible?

As a child I found it hard to put the pieces together because something did not ring true. It was not until I married Christopher that I learned another way of looking at the Christian texts that seem to promote the idea of a judgemental and punishing God. Christopher spent five years studying texts in Greek, Latin and Hebrew. His main source for reference was a great tome with the New Testament text down the left hand side of the page and columns giving the Greek translation alongside, then the Latin and lastly the Hebrew. Hearing the different versions was fascinating and illuminating, but over and over he would say: "This is not original; this was added in the fourth century." I was astonished because I had always assumed that the Bible text was absolutely authentic. I found it very unsettling and wanted to know what proof there was for what he was saying.

I remember one day he was showing me a familiar passage from the third chapter of St John's Gospel, where Jesus tells Nicodemus that he must be born again to enter into the Kingdom of God. Nicodemus questions the idea of entering into his mother's womb a second time to be reborn. Christopher told me that when you looked at the Greek and the Hebrew side by side, you knew it was a later addition. The word for 'born again' in Greek means two things: to be 'from above' or to be 'born again' physically. But there is only one word in Hebrew: to be 'from above'. Jesus and Nicodemus were Jews and spoke Aramaic. In that language there would be no concept of entering into a mother's womb and being born again in a practical sense. Such a conversation just would not take place. But in Greek it makes perfect sense. "So you see," Christopher told me, "scholars know that this was originally written in Greek, and quite a lot later, probably in the fourth century. Jesus wrote nothing down. The gospels' accounts were spoken and passed around person to person. Nothing was written down until forty to seventy years later. The language they were finally written down in was Greek. There were lots of other 'gospels' that didn't make it when they finally put together what became known as the New Testament in the fourth century, and by then the Church was formed and was trying to heavily influence what people believed and understood. So the words 'born again', in Greek, did not come from Jesus's mouth, but from fourth century Christian leaders. The Church was now teaching that humanity was inherently sinful and needed to be redeemed – that salvation had to be earned.

This was a great surprise to me, but it at last explained the discordant note that creeps into the texts as you read what we are told Jesus said and did. The fourth century was a violent time and Christianity was spreading like wildfire. Control and direction were clearly needed and systems had to be put in place to make sure that people believed what was becoming the orthodox message of the Church. Texts that were not approved by the Church were declared to be heretical and burned; people were likewise also being destroyed for taking a different view. So we see a victory for fear and control.

Jesus gave one big commandment: "Love one another as I have loved you." This is a message of transcendence – something we can choose to do for ourselves. How different the world would have been had this self-empowering message dominated Church teaching.

Ancient stories also abounded around the concept of the father sacrificing his first born (Abraham and Isaac) and in the early years after the resurrection people believed that they were living in 'the end time' when judgement would befall the earth and the elect would be saved. Any and all means were to be employed to save people from the retribution that was to come. Thus, instead of Jesus bringing good news of transcendence through Divine Love, he became the Saviour Judge and a theology of sin, guilt and damnation tied the New Testament to the Old. The judging Christ replaced the forgiving, uplifting Jesus.

The leading figure in this movement was St Paul, who used his great intellect to change the compassionate message that Jesus had taught to one of salvation only by faith in the death and resurrection of Jesus. Recognising the divinity of Jesus from his rising from the dead, Paul taught this doctrine as a means of escaping judgement and the wrath to come. Paul, of course, had not lived with Jesus and did not have the benefit of the four Gospels that were written after his death. He had a vision and an experience of the post-resurrection risen Christ, but did not know the whole story as we do. Thus grew up a bewildering theology of story and myth for two thousand years, which included the subjugation of women and the much-feared coming judgement. How could something so beautiful and full of promise become so distorted?

In many, sometimes desperate, conversations with Christopher we went over and over the subject of how it could be that we knew Jesus in our hearts and in our lives as a loving and protective presence, and felt his spirit surrounding us like a cocoon of nurturing love, and yet looming over the history of our faith was violence and intolerance. It felt like a burden too great to be borne and it was not something that could be shared with those around us; we had no desire to undermine people's traditional faith and belief as it was clearly very precious to them and a great comfort especially in times of need. Tim also felt that it was important not to unsettle the people we were ministering to. When Bishop John Robinson had courageously published *Honest to God*[12] back in 1963, saying some of these things, all hell broke loose in the Church and he resigned as Bishop of Woolwich and went back to academia. Later on Bishop John Spong in America was similarly placed, producing a number of challenging books, and referring to himself as a Christian in exile.

In the light of all this, how strange that we personally could continue to experience a constant and blissful spiritual energy that surrounded us and lit up everything that we did. Our children absorbed it in their early years through the nightly prayers and hymns that we shared even when they were too young to understand. As adults they still speak of the enormous comfort they received at the end of our evening ritual as Christopher made the sign of the cross on each little forehead and solemnly pronounced:

> *Into the Lord's most gracious mercy and protection I commit you.*
> *May the Lord bless you and keep you,*
> *May the Lord make his face to shine upon you*
> *And be gracious unto you.*
> *May the Lord lift up the light of his countenance upon you*
> *And give you peace*
> *Now and forever more. Amen*

Did any of it make sense to their little minds? Perhaps not, but it spoke to something deep and profound within them. They have passed it on to their children for the same reason. Family traditions and rituals are very powerful. They form the scaffolding and structure upon which we build our lives when we in turn become independent.

We were finding in our anxiety about Penny, her approaching mastectomy and all the fears that the diagnosis of cancer brought, that the scaffolding of our developing spiritual life sustained us through the valley of the shadow of death, as well as the joyous uplands of communion with the Divine.

Chapter 6
The Birth of the Bristol Cancer Help Centre

Penny said of her first hospital stay in Bath that being on her own there while awaiting surgery actually allowed her time to think. She went over the sorrows of her last months, the loss of her parents and the heavy weeks of bereavement, and slowly thoughts began to form in her mind. She had not been herself since their death. Nothing was the same. Could it be also true that things had changed physically in her body, as well as in how she felt?

Penny had a thorough background in Chinese medicine as well as in acupuncture, and as a therapist she always took into account what was going on in people's lives before and at the time of their illness. Now she put her skills to use to think about her own body. Had months of low spirits reduced the ability of her immune system to protect her from cancer? Could there be a connection? The more she chased the thoughts around her mind, the more sense it made.

Penny shared her thoughts with some of her visitors and their main response was to encourage her to get on with the mastectomy and then look at the psychology later. In interviews with medical staff Penny put forward her new found thoughts, but was greeted with incomprehension. They also said such things could wait until later and surgery was arranged. But this was eating away at Penny's mind – so much so that she soon announced that she was postponing the surgery while she went home to think more clearly what she should do. All the power of the medical team was brought to bear on changing her mind, but in the end she prevailed. Promising to return soon, she managed to get herself home.

Tim, Christopher and I joined her as soon as possible to give healing and support. The two priests stood either side of her and I knelt at her feet, holding her hands. She was shaking and desperate. Even without treatment, hospital had been a hard experience for her. The healing began and deepened into a powerful energy that we could all feel. Slowly Penny stopped shaking and began to enter a deep meditative calm. Half an hour passed before Tim gave a blessing and we all relaxed. Colour had returned to Penny's face and she turned to us and said, "Now I know what to do."

A friend had been telling Penny of a clinic in Bavaria run by a Dr Josef Issels, who had an alternative and new approach to treating cancer. He was having some success but what he was doing was very controversial. Penny thought her next step was to go for a consultation and an opinion. I never heard what her husband David thought about this but, desperate with worry, he agreed to fly with her to Munich and visit the clinic to hear what Dr Issels had to say.

Dr Issels asked Penny, "Do you know why you have cancer?" and with tears falling she told him of her parents' death. He said, "That is the key you must turn in the lock," and he went on to describe how he could help her with his alternative medical treatments. So Penny decided to stay and David returned alone. Desperately worried for Penny, for their three small children, and for himself in having to cope with so much, David busied himself putting all Penny's belongings into a suitcase so that she had what she needed for an extended stay in Germany. I offered to carry the case to Penny and to stay with her.

It was there, just a few weeks later, in her little room by a lake in Bavaria that together we dreamed up what was to become the Bristol Cancer Help Centre, later to be called Penny Brohn Cancer Care.

Penny had been very certain about what she was doing to start with but, by the time I got there, she had lived through several lonely days and was ready to weep her tears. I remembered hearing Dr Elizabeth Kubler-Ross, that great pioneer of the hospice movement, say that each of us carries a bucket of tears inside us. Penny's bucket was overflowing now that she had someone sympathetic at her side. As she wept, she said that she could only do so because we were far from home and there was no one to distress. "It would upset the children too much," she said. And I thought of how we are constantly handling and adapting our behaviour so that no one is upset. "We," Penny said, meaning people with cancer, "need a safe place in order to do this." Providing a safe place was uppermost in her mind, and in the decades that have followed it has been one of the most powerful things that we have done for people in crisis.

· · · · · · ·

We all need a safe place to process the vagaries of life. Something that we profoundly need is missing from our lives if we are constantly surrounded by activity and noise. Life, in the past, built in these spaces. To get anywhere, it was necessary to walk. Without artificial light, our ancestors sat in the gloom and slept in the dark. Food was cultivated, animals milked and fish tempted out of the streams. All around the stuff of daily life lay a profound silence and people matched the beating of their hearts to it. It was cold and uncomfortable of course, but I feel it must be true that, within, each person had more space. Ritual and religion may have been considered opium for the masses but it served a purpose beyond the obvious and comforted many a sorrowing heart. Life that always ended in death had a pattern to it, and was seen as a preparation for what was to come. People didn't want to live and then depart this earth as if their lives had no significance so they believed that every day was a preparation for what was to come, if they were to take the whole of their soul energy with them as they departed.

Family ties and shared belief also provided meaning and purpose to each short and difficult life. As we dismiss the old practices as ignorant superstition, we possibly miss what it was that they did for communities. Those practices and religious observances served to hold together people who otherwise might have had very separate lives.

These are profound thoughts. I find it puzzling to know where we can go in today's life to find the space and silence and the resolve to take such disturbing notions of our own mortality out of their wrappings and look at them. Death today always comes as a shock. People say the notion of dying has taken them by surprise. Even if we believe that something survives death, holding a belief is not the same as maintaining a practice that will act as a bridge to carry us forward when the time comes. There was a time when such soul preparation was integral to people's lives but now, having abandoned religious practice, we have to create space and time for this sort of consideration. If we do so we begin to realise that dying was considered not an ending but a transition to a different form of life.

Elizabeth Kubler-Ross, in her book *On Life after Death*[13], recounts her near-death experience saying that, on leaving the physical body in death, you float through a tunnel, pass through a gate or cross a bridge. "Having been born in Switzerland," she says, "I was allowed to cross a pass in the Alps covered with wild flowers. Everyone is met by the Heaven he or she imagines and I was allowed to experience this transition by crossing a mountain pass of incomparable beauty." Dr Kubler-Ross returned from her near-death experience with vivid memories and transformed herself in preparation for the work that she was going to do. Her story exactly mirrored that of Tim Tiley, whose own story of a near-death experience began our awakening to the ministry of healing.

Kubler-Ross's journey beyond the death of the body continues with a description of an ineffable light that then surrounded and embraced her. This is the light of love, and she says.

> *After seeing the light, no one wants to go back. In this light you will experience what man could have been. Here there is understanding without judging, here you experience unconditional love. You come to know that all your life on earth was nothing but a school that you had to go through in order to pass certain tests and learn special lessons. As soon as you have finished this school and mastered your lessons, you are allowed to go home, to graduate.*

In her many books and lectures, Dr Kubler-Ross deals with the most difficult questions such as why do dear little children have to die? Her answer was quite simple, if controversial nowadays: "They have learned in a very short period what each has to learn, which could be different things for different people." The one thing we all have to learn is the practice of unconditional love and that points us to the great teachings of Jesus: "Love one another as I have loved you." Loving action comes from a loving heart, and that is our task: to choose love in the face of fear, compassion in the face of self-absorption, and hope in the face of despair.

• • • • • • •

I was with Penny for some of the nine weeks that she spent at Issel's clinic, and we talked more and more about the impact of cancer as a form of awakening to the journey of the soul. She herself became more positive and cheerful as the naturopathic treatments began to have a positive effect. Her tumour was shrinking and her energy was rising. With increasing enthusiasm we began planning what we could take back to Bristol from all the things we were learning, and how some form of help could be given to people with cancer through our healing centre. It was interesting to see how planning for the future brought colour to Penny's cheeks and light to her eyes. There seemed to be an association between her passion for something and an increased vitality.

As we planned we realised we would need a doctor in the driving seat if we were extending our healing work in Bristol to concentrate on the particular needs of people with cancer. Penny was sure it was a legal requirement. I was totally ignorant about such things, but wanting to encourage Penny I said I was sure we would find one. This touched a nerve. "Would I be sitting here in Germany if there had been even one doctor like Issels in England?" she exploded. "There isn't one! Not one." But in fact there was.

When I flew back to Bristol for Christopher's birthday celebrations in October 1979, there was a letter awaiting me from a vicar we knew who lived in Shropshire. He had visited our healing centre the year before and was writing to us to ask if we could help a doctor friend of his called Alec Forbes who wanted to launch a pilot scheme to try a new approach to the treatment of cancer. I couldn't believe my eyes. Here was a letter, written in Shropshire to us in Bristol, about a doctor in Plymouth who exactly fitted what we had been imagining in Germany! My head was spinning and again I faced the question: who took the message? How was it that our prayer was answered in such a complete and immediate way? Except that we hadn't actually been praying, we had been focusing on the need for a doctor and exclaiming that we needed someone like Dr Issels in England. This was divine guidance and couldn't be ignored.

Only many years later did I again realise the power of intention: the focused thought of the mind allied to a powerful surge of the heart. This had happened before when we wanted schools for our children in Bristol and lived 100 miles away.

Dr Alec Forbes was a senior consultant physician at Plymouth General Hospital. He was approaching retirement and was very fed up with his routine work. When we met just before Christmas in 1979 he told us sadly that it was as if patients didn't want to heal themselves, they just wanted to be given pills. However, he had observed that people faced by the crisis of cancer were prepared to change in order to overcome their disease. He found them a pleasure to work with because they were open to try anything and were focused on helping themselves. He had been studying what was happening in clinics around the world and was desperate to try things for himself.

By the time Penny was home again, also shortly before Christmas 1979, her tumour had apparently disappeared and she had no need for the mastectomy. Family reunions and Christmas stockings took priority, but early in 1980 Dr Forbes came to present his ideas at a talk at the healing centre. It was then that he offered to help us launch our new adventure. The thing we had been talking endlessly about in Germany was about to happen: we were going to devote our work at the healing centre to the particular needs of people with cancer and we had a doctor - a senior consultant physician, no less. We had no money to pay him, of course, but he made light of that. We opened our doors to the first clients in October of that year, with Alec as our first medical director. We renamed the healing centre The Bristol Cancer Help Centre.

There was so much to learn. We gathered all the books we could find and passed them round so that all our healers and clients could read them. We attended seminars, conferences and lectures and began to meet many others out there who were passionately connecting to the interface of body, mind, emotions and spirit. And we had imagined we were alone! We met people like Beata Bishop who had used Gerson therapy to heal her cancer; she had a German background and combined old naturopathic therapy with western medicine and was many years into remission.

So much was happening and of course we were trying to keep the 'day job' going because there was no thought of charging people for our services. A rota of volunteers who believed in what we were doing offered to cook, clean, answer phones and keep records and the only charge we made was £1 for lunch. Slowly we developed an ongoing programme that included group work and individual appointments with a doctor, counsellor, healer, nutritionist and massage therapist. For the first year or so we worked only one day a week, but soon it was clear that that was not enough, and it extended to two, then three. The number of people seeking our help increased week by week. The word was spreading.

In December 1982 Prince Charles made a seminal speech to the British Medical Association. According to Jonathan Dimbleby's biography *The Prince of Wales*[14], neither advisors nor specialists were involved in the composition of the speech, but only, as the Prince would say, 'my intuition'. It was the 150th anniversary of the foundation of the BMA and His Royal Highness was president for that special year. He set about telling the doctors that science had become 'estranged from nature'. He said the doctor should have "the intuition which is necessary to understand the patient, his body, his disease. He must have the feel and the touch that makes it possible for him to be in sympathetic communication with the patient's spirits... the good doctor's therapeutic success largely depends on his ability to inspire the patient with confidence and to mobilise his will to health..." The Prince went on to urge that the deep communication of healing should be reincorporated into the practice of medicine.

Dimbleby said: "The vivid imagery and the radical thrust of his words sent a shudder through the medical establishment, both the practitioners and their symbiotic partners in the drug industry... in July he heaped fuel on the fire by accepting an invitation to open the Bristol Cancer Help Centre, which had been running for three years."

Indeed the Prince did!

Our work had grown to such an extent that we had completely

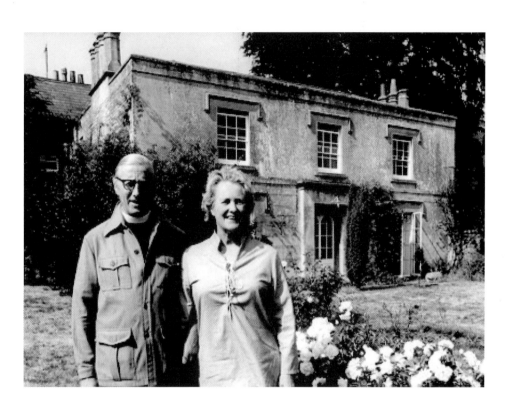

Tim and Mystica Tiley outside the Old Rectory

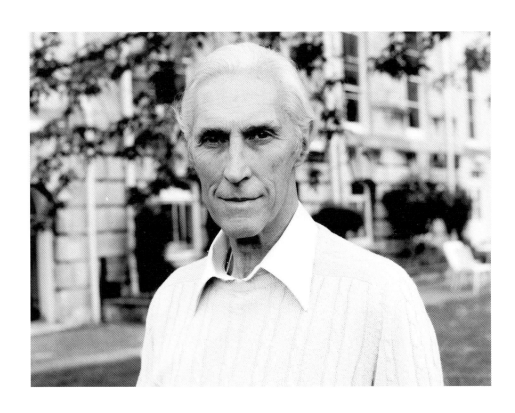

Dr Alec Forbes outside Grove House

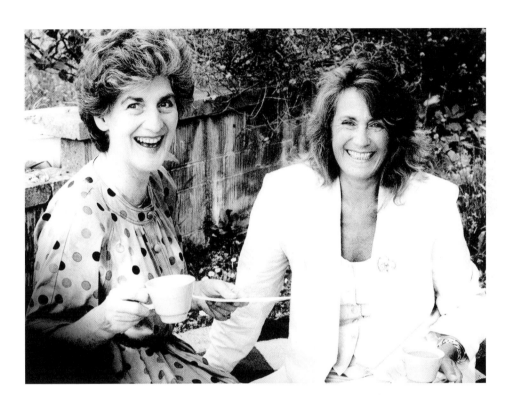

Pat with Penny Brohn

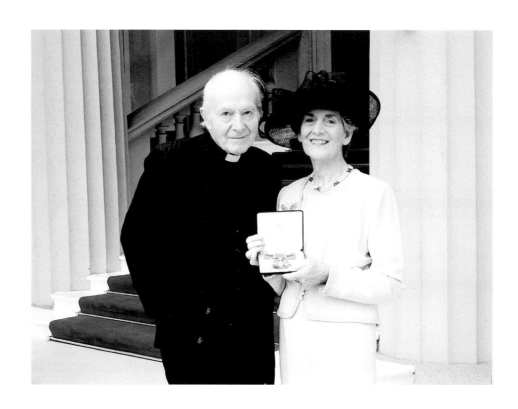

Pat receiving her MBE, with Christopher

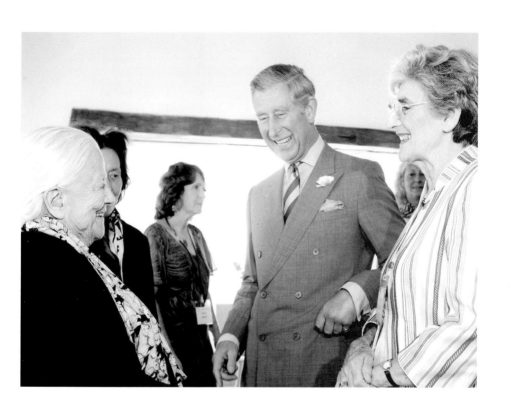

Pat with His Royal Highness The Prince of Wales,
at the opening of Ham Green House

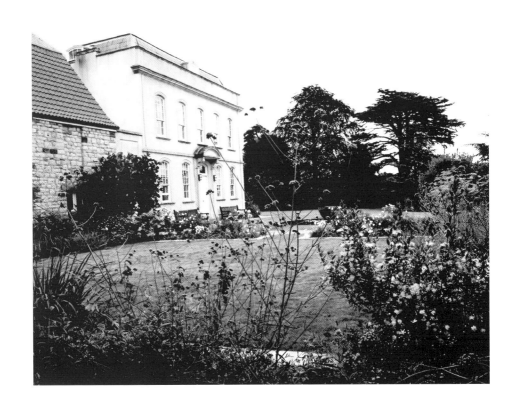

Penny Brohn Cancer Care Centre, as it is today

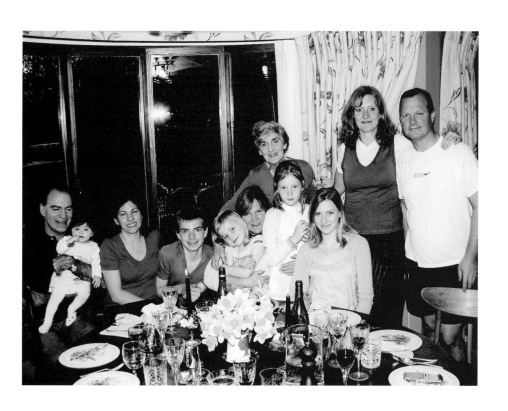

Surrounded by her family: children, children-in-law, and grandchildren. Pat's son John is behind the lens.

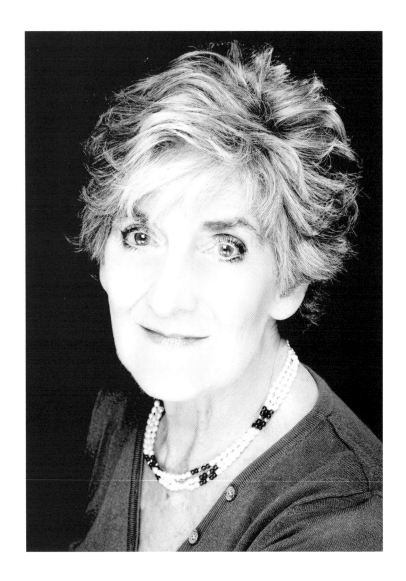

The late Pat Pilkington, MBE
3rd November 1928 -19th August 2013

outgrown our private house and we had started to look for suitable premises in which to run a full-time and residential centre. The few country houses that we inspected were completely hopeless, and then a former convent in the heart of Clifton in Bristol came on the market. It was hugely expensive and we had no money. However, when Christopher approached the bank a loan was agreed, with our family home as security. Every developer in Bristol was after this highly desirable property but, in what seemed to us truly a miracle, we secured the property against all this competition and completed on the purchase in the autumn of 1982, just before Prince Charles made his momentous speech to the BMA.

As soon as we heard reports of the Prince's address to the medical establishment we wrote to St James's Palace telling His Royal Highness that we completely fulfilled his profile of care and described our work. Great excitement followed when a letter came from the Palace asking for a visit. Weeks went by as they struggled with an over full royal diary, and then the idea grew that this could become a more public occasion if the Prince would officially open our new premises in Clifton. Thus it was that a close and supportive relationship came about that some years later grew into royal patronage.

What had we taken on? We had no money and no income. We had none of the skills required to run what in effect was to become a hotel with therapeutic services - a business. What sort of madness had possessed us to hand the deeds of our own home as well as the new 'clinic' over to the bank as collateral? How were we to acquire the skills of fundraising in double quick time and, indeed, when our work was so innovative, how was even the most skilled of fundraisers to appeal to a public that could not understand what it was we were doing?

Was it the ultimate folly to believe in the intuitive guidance that had got us this far? As always we turned to Tim Tiley, who told us it was all part of a plan and that we should hold our nerve and not give way to fear. We sometimes thought that we had not known the smell and taste of fear until then and, as Penny had been forced to open her eyes to the diagnosis of cancer, we now had to learn how to walk with fear and be unafraid. It was easier said than done.

Chapter 7
Spiritual Work with Clients

For Christopher and I, and for others of our core team involved in this hugely risky adventure, being with Tim brought back our sense of proportion. He told us that in life there are no guarantees and we had to choose love over fear. We were not here trying to transform the world single-handed. As we later read in Emmanuel, from the viewpoint of fear, no guarantee would be big and strong enough; from the viewpoint of love, no guarantee was necessary. We were a powerful group with an even more powerful idea. But, Tim said, the beginning of this transformation rested with each one of us. "When your heart is open you are in truth. Remember the spiritual being that you essentially are. When you know you are connected to all the power in the universe then you can do what Jesus taught: you can move mountains."

It was astonishing how courage returned when we sat talking to Tim. He had a direct line of guidance into his consciousness that had been with him ever since his boyhood experience of near-death. This profoundly life-changing event, in which he got his 'head into heaven', shaped everything that followed. He had the gift of being able to tune in to the higher realm and get answers to his questions. On our behalf he asked if what we were doing was what was needed, and he was told all was well and we must hold the vision and have no fear. It is impossible to exaggerate what a help it was to us all to be able to confirm our own intuitive feelings in this way. As we went back to struggle with all the many problems that threatened to engulf us, we held in mind the concept that this frightening situation was there in our lives to make us develop skills and abilities that we never knew we had.

Penny kept increasing in health and maintained Issel's programme of therapeutic support. A healthy vegetarian dairy-free diet was supplemented by fresh juices and vitamins and it was obviously having a powerful effect. She also meditated and spent time in counselling and healing; she knew that she had had a narrow escape and was happy to work at all levels of body, mind, emotions and spirit to restore wellbeing. "Traditional Chinese medicine considers cancer a disease like any other: the body is out of balance and restoring balance requires a lot of attention," she told us. It was a powerful lesson to those of us who took our health for granted.

Penny was a wonderful inspiration to all our clients and visitors. She was truly able to say to clients, "I know what you are going through," as she held out loving arms to them.

Prince Charles opened Grove House on July 15, 1983. During a two-hour visit he spent time talking to the doctors and watching a relaxation class. He took part in a biofeedback session with Alec Forbes and chatted with clients. It was a huge honour, and a wonderful confirmation of the value of our work.

Soon after we moved to Grove House we were able to take on our first residential clients to join our day clients. Slowly we assembled a marvellous team of staff, and of course we had to pay them. Money was a constant problem and Christopher often had to use his personal skills to persuade the bank to keep up our loan. Reluctantly we had to begin to make a charge for our services, and redoubled our efforts in learning how to fundraise.

In 1984, after fourteen years in the City Parish ministry, Christopher took early retirement and moved his office into the Centre to concentrate on the healing ministry, as well as head up the fundraising department. We moved out of the rectory in Bristol into our cottage in the Mendip Hills, now beautifully restored. We found living in the country an unexpected delight, even though we now had to commute to the Centre.

Once Christopher had settled into his new role he found that at last he was in his element. As he quietly chatted to clients in the chapel preparing to give them healing, he found a spiritual depth that had been mostly missing in his work for the Church. He became much less careworn and a great deal happier, and felt that at last he was where he should be. He was living the way of the heart: he was in his truth. Unconstrained by formal church services, he was able to bring a new level of spirituality and awakened to a reality beyond the five senses and the things of ordinary life. He was able to suggest that to ask for actual physical proof of a purely spiritual dimension of existence is a contradiction of terms. You have to see 'through' not 'with' the eye. Where are the boundaries between the seen and the unseen world, he would ponder. What is it that we feel when we are surrounded by a presence in a bluebell wood in springtime? What is it that comes to us in a phrase of music, or the cadence in a line of poetry?

Some people responded more sensitively to such thoughts than others. Celia had come to Bristol at regular intervals from her council flat in the East End of London. She had been told she had three months to live, and had refused the treatment offered by her hospital. She had heard about us on the radio and had insisted on coming, although we were full and had no appointments. Christopher made time to see her and was the first to hear her story. She had nursed her husband through a long cancer journey and found herself bankrupt and alone after he was gone. She ignored her own symptoms until it was too late, and all she wanted to do was die. "That was, until they told me at the hospital that I would die in three months. Then I wanted to live," she explained.

During the healing session it was clear that Celia was highly sensitive and she began to see angelic beings in the chapel. During the days that followed she threw herself into every aspect of the healing programme and went home armed with a great deal of information, a bag of vitamins and the picture she had painted in art therapy. A great golden sun hung in a blue sky and Celia told us that she was going to imagine her tumour as a block of ice which the sun would gradually melt as she held the image in mind day after day. How could something so simple work? Or was it the healing, or the nutritious wholefood diet that she embraced excitedly?

Week after week she took the train from Paddington and came to see us in Bristol looking astonishingly good for someone who was in her last weeks. Something had changed significantly in Celia's life, and in her body. She would never let anyone examine her, so we never knew, but the three months passed and then three more, and by then she was running a support group in her area of London. She continued to join us week by week because she always wanted healing from Christopher, and she found a useful role for herself in encouraging new clients to work with the 'Bristol programme', as our whole therapeutic approach had by now become labelled. I think Celia opened her heart and embraced life once again when she found the Bristol Cancer Help Centre. Everything changed for her and I remember her saying, "I never knew birds sang in the winter, until I had cancer."

This perfect, clear perception is the way the heart sees. It takes a leap of faith to shift our focus from the mind, the brain and intellect, in order to enter the spaciousness of the heart. There are no boundaries here; when we love, we find we can love more. Indeed the joy of falling in love is that suddenly we are in love with life, as well as the beloved. Everything shimmers and sparkles as our hearts radiate a powerful field of electromagnetic energy: a measurable field of high vibration. "Even recalling an event of love or joy through creative imagination throws out a high-frequency bridge from the pre-frontal cortex to the limbic-heart system," says Joseph Chiltern Pearce in *The Biology of Transcendence*[15]. "The heart automatically reciprocates on that same frequency, lifting us to a higher level, opening an order of functioning not available to either intellect or imagination alone. It is our ability to transcend, to go beyond limitation and restraint, and it is our biological birthright. Transcendence is the central theme of Jesus's teaching."

The heart then is far more than the pump that keeps life pulsing within us. The metaphysical heart receives life energy, prana, chi, ki – whatever you may like to call it – that is spiritual energy flowing in the universe. It fills us with universal wisdom and it connects us to all that is, human and divine, in the world of nature and in the realms of the stars.

When we have opened our heart sufficiently to let life energy flow we can allow the start of a healing process. Our life journey could be imagined as a canoe ride on a river, sometimes peacefully flowing and sometimes turbulent. The scenery may stretch out on either side in vistas of calm meadows and gentle hills, and sometimes we seem to have reversed the direction of the little craft as we paddle for dear life upstream against the current. Much of what we have been taught in our culture and in our education is like paddling upstream.

Have we not been dismayed and exhausted in the struggle to conform to what others want us to be? As I write this a vivid picture comes unbidden before my mind's eye: I am a new mother and my baby of a few months continues to cry as I try to settle and resettle him in his cot for the night. Never short of advisors in my vicarage home, I am told that I must shut the door and let him cry. "He's got to learn," they said. The anguish of listening to his cries still brings tears all these years later. He did learn, of course, but at what cost? That felt like paddling upstream, and my trembling heart knew it then and knows it still.

I repeat the question: at what cost have we followed our culture of stiff upper lip, of doing what is expected of us and ignoring our heart's code? We have paid the price in many, many ways and each of us will have an individual story. The awakening that we speak of is coming to see with new eyes the eyes of the heart. Our heart knows who we are and knows our purpose in coming into this life. We are surrounded by grace and the essence of grace is unconditional love. As we awaken to our own personal divinity we are able to see the path before us more clearly. Knowing that we do not walk alone encourages us to keep connected and to move forward with joy and courage.

Looking back at my life with Christopher, wonderful as it has been, I see how things were in the vicarage at Bromsgrove in the 1960s. We had a new baby and two small children and at times it was like paddling upstream. We were at everyone's beck and call, constantly with 'open house', people coming and going and absolutely no privacy. But Christopher had a way of seeing with the heart and after a year or so he hit on the brilliant idea of putting our caravan in a woodland caravan site about forty minutes from home. It was a wonderful place and completely deserted mid-week. So he and I would try every so often to sneak off there for a little time alone. I used to complain, "When God is your boss, there is no end to the demand that is put upon you," and he would shut my grumbling mouth with a kiss and help me to make the most of the precious moments.

That struggle we had with our fragmented life in the vicarage was as nothing to the stories we were to hear later from clients coming to the Bristol Cancer Help Centre. I vividly recall meeting Gabby for the first time. She was young and beautiful, with a warm Scottish lilt and a compelling way of speaking. When it was her turn to tell her story she let out an expletive and said she was absolutely furious with the consultant at her hospital. "He just sat there looking down at his hands that were clasped together on the desk in front of him. The papers with the results of my scan were underneath them," she said, "and he slowly began to tell me that what had appeared as an operable condition was actually terminally spread, and that I had only weeks to live. For a moment I couldn't take it in, and then I was filled with this great ball of anger and I leaned forward and took his clasped hands in mine and shouted at him. I banged his hands up and down as I ranted on. I shouted that we didn't have two lovely children for me to go and die on them at junior school. 'No!' I bellowed. 'I am going to live until I see them right the way through their new school.'" Gabby paused for a moment and then went on quietly "Do you know, he just let me hit him and shout at him, and he just sat there saying 'I'm sorry'."

We were all mesmerised by her story and many people said how they wished they had had the courage to do the same, and express their anger. I heard Gabby tell that story again and again over the months and years, and she did live to see her children through school. What none of us had the sense to suggest to her was that she should extend her intention. We should have put into her mind that she would live to see them graduate from university, get married, have grandchildren and so on. The strange and extraordinary thing is this: almost to the day when the second child left school, Gabby's symptoms returned and in a couple of months she was gone. She had kept her promise, and how we regretted not having the wisdom to help her reframe her goal. What was at work? Is it some sort of destiny, or do we underestimate the extraordinary power of fear and negative expectation?

Chapter 8
Love and Fear

Fear is a great teacher as long as we know how to use it. I have a book on my shelf called *Feel the Fear and Do it Anyway* by Susan Jeffers[16]. In it she says the trick is to make the situation work for you rather than allow it to incapacitate you. We all know about 'fight or flight' and the adrenalin rush that makes extraordinary things occur. It may be because something like this was happening to us in our work that we became so active, creative and extraordinarily positive. Not, I hasten to say, that anything was easy, but it was amazing how what we needed seemed to come to hand in so many strange and diverse ways.

Being part of a group most certainly helped; alone we might individually have gone in to frightened rabbit mode, frozen in each situation, but together we felt strong. At the time it was exciting and immensely fulfilling, yet looking back I wonder how we found the courage to do what we did. As we began to see the life and the light coming back into clients' lives, we knew we were on the right road.

It was a tremendous help to have residential accommodation and be there every day of the week. The clients in turn picked up the creative magic and opened their own homes to start the first cancer support groups all around the country. Indeed, as time passed and we became more aware of the potential everyone carried within themselves, it became more and more obvious that we all carry this amazing ability to teach and to pass on our experience and knowledge. Could it be that the unwelcome wake-up call that comes into people's lives with the diagnosis of cancer is a way of summoning up the teacher within that lies dormant until released by the energy surrounding the crisis?

When the Children of Israel were travelling for forty years through the wilderness to get to the Promised Land, they were given manna to eat. They were told that it could not be stored. They had to take enough for each day to keep them going, and then go out and gather it afresh the next day. It is the same with choosing love over fear. It has to be done every day. It cannot be stored. A daily practice of prayer, meditation and mindfulness is required so that fear doesn't creep in by the back door.

Mindfulness is another way of talking about being connected to the Divinity within. We didn't have mobile phones at this time, but had we known about them we might have described it as always being in touch with God, as if He were constantly on the end of the line. And the strange thing is that we actually felt as if someone was there, real or imagined, and that sense of being connected, that sense of the Golden Thread, was enough just to see us through each day.

I look back and ask myself how real this sense of connection to the Divine really was, and now with hindsight I can say that I don't think it matters. If it was real enough to be helpful, it was real enough! Perhaps we make too much of proof and scientific reality, when all we actually need for a day's journey is enough to see us through in good heart. I feel that this is nearer to the teaching of Jesus and Buddha than the dogma, beliefs and creeds that have caused so much bloodshed over the centuries. And maybe this is why in both the Old Testament and the New there are so many injunctions to 'fear not'. The bigger the task the more focused we have to be. Practising with the small things in life is preparation for the great mountains that we sometimes have to climb.

It was the small things that I first noticed about Douglas. He was quite ill with bowel cancer that had spread to many of his bones, but he was perfectly upright and vigorous. He was elderly and had the neat bearing of a former military man. The shine on his polished brown shoes spoke of the careful attention he gave every detail. He was very neat in his dress, and his piercing blue eyes lit up when he smiled. Once his shyness had worn off, he never stopped talking, and with his Scottish accent and humour, he was great company. He came regularly and we all got very fond of him, fond enough to greet him with a hug and a kiss on the cheek.

We soon began to notice that he was arriving earlier and earlier, and that he made his entrance slowly going from volunteers to staff embracing each one, and making cheery conversation. "You only come to see us for the kisses," announced one of the staff in reception, and Douglas immediately admitted how he adored the warm welcome we all gave him.

Slowly, over many conversations and counselling sessions, it became clear that this affectionate and warm-hearted man had a home life that was barren and without affection. He always came on his own. Douglas told us that his monthly visits to Bristol kept the rest of his life going. He practised relaxation and meditation daily, and did his best with the diet. All in all he kept surprisingly well over several years in spite of a very poor prognosis. We used to have regular meetings with the full staff group to share our different perspectives on the progress of our clients and we all began to think that the attention he enjoyed with us, and the affection he received was somehow lifting his spirits sufficiently to keep him going.

Tim Tiley always said love was the great healer. "Jesus had one simple message: love God and love your neighbour", and here we could see that even a simple affectionate and loving attitude on the part of all the staff affected Douglas so much. It also built up a warm and caring atmosphere in the building that people remarked on as they came in the door. Celia, whose psychic gifts had returned now that she was well and happy, said that the whole place was full of angels. How I wished I could see them!

We grew busier and busier and sometimes wondered what our true purpose was. "Should we be trying to bring people to God?" I asked Tim. "Good heavens, no," he exclaimed. "There isn't time for that - people are only here for a week. No," he urged us, "tell them that death isn't the end. No one dies; we just slip from one reality to another, in and out of both sides of life. Then there will be time to come to know God. And they will."

Listening to Tim speaking with full conviction and knowledge, I had no idea that he himself was nearing the end of his own life. If I had known, I would have asked a great many more questions and spent more time in his company. But he was vigorous and well and such thoughts never occurred to us. Then, in 1985, just two weeks from apparent health and vigour, his life came to an end leaving his family and all of us absolutely and totally bereft. He had died of double pneumonia. Penny wept for all the healing sessions she could have had and had postponed. I wept for the unanswered questions that I had not thought to ask. Christopher, as he took Tim's funeral, spread his hands towards the crowded congregation and asked "Whose hands now will give the healing?" and he invited everyone there to pick up Tim's mantle and reach out in healing to the world. He had taught us so much. All the work that we were now doing had its origins in Tim's teaching. He had held and guided us through the early years, when it was all so new and frightening.

There is a memorial stone to Tim on the wall of Litton Church on which are inscribed the words 'Priest, healer and friend', and the quote 'Put love first'.

Now he was gone we were going to have to stand on our own feet. It was a bleak prospect in spite of the fact that the work was going very well. All we could think of at that funeral service was that we could have made more of the opportunities that had been ours, and now 'time like an ever rolling stream' had borne one of its sons away, leaving us absolutely bereft. We knew we needed to remain strong, yet we felt far from courageous in that bleak moment.

I could hear Tim's voice in my head giving the instruction: "Tell them that death is not the end." More and more it seemed to me that all the essential things that we were doing in teaching healthy lifestyle and nutrition and offering counselling and healing, were taking people only so far. Of course, the progress people made was highly significant and it was clear that having some means of improving their health gave people a tremendous sense that they could help themselves, and that they were not helpless.

Yet some people seemed to move on ahead of this into spiritual enquiry. Many returned to the church, chapel, synagogue or mosque of their upbringing, so finding nourishment for their souls. Others began intense spiritual enquiry that seemed to go beyond particular faiths, into a oneness that embraced all.

I was touched to find a relevant quotation from Florence Nightingale. Although she was deeply religious, she was extremely tolerant and honoured the beliefs, rituals and practices of all cultures she met under the British Empire. Her embrace of cultural diversity was ahead of its time and is particularly apparent in her forty years work to improve conditions in India. She stressed that all the world's great religions should be studied because, as she put it, this gave "unity to the whole – one continuous thread of interest to all these pearls".

To see the diversity of religions as pearls strung along the thread of spirituality makes sense as long as you can see each expression of faith as valid for the person involved. If we take a view that there is only one right way to righteousness, then we are immediately into problems. It was such conviction, of course, that led to cries of heresy in the past, to the Inquisition and other horrors.

I recall Tim telling us that the way to God is always through the heart, and that we have a divine energy within our hearts that is able to recognise and relate to God. In this way it may be true to say that Christians come to God through Christ - through the divine part of us that incarnated as a spiral of God Energy. Someone like Jesus was completely filled with Christ Energy, which is why he could heal and perform miracles. We have the same potential, depending on how 'filled' we are in our turn. Jesus always said that if faith and belief were equally present his followers could do what he did and even greater things.

What we see in the life of Jesus is that he always chose love, not fear. He taught with love and compassion; he healed the sick and fed the hungry. He knew that death was only a door into the next reality and spoke of his Father's house having many mansions. "If it were not so," he said, "would I have told you that I go to prepare a place for you, where I will receive you unto myself?" When he faced his accusers, he chose love in his silent response. When they crucified him he prayed, "Father forgive them; they know not what they do." On the cross he promised the dying thief, "Today you will be with me in paradise." He looked down from the cross in loving concern to his mother and the disciple whom he loved, and commended them to each other. His final words to God were: "Father, into thy hands I commend my spirit."

At each point in the desolate journey he chose love, not fear. It is recorded that the centurion in charge of the execution was so impressed with his demeanour that he said, "Truly this was a son of God." Perfect love casts out fear, as we are told, and this is the choice we face day by day in our lesser Calvaries. It is an awesome task, but made easier for someone in a Christian tradition in every moment by asking the question "What would Jesus do now?" before making our choice for love.

• • • • • • •

We mourned Tim's passing in every sort of way. He had always been there and was endlessly ready to give us encouragement and guidance. Tim had appeared in our lives like a beacon of light with his ability to heal and his stories of the next world and his near-death experience. We had learnt from him and the result had been our extraordinary cancer centre that was growing in strength day by day. Because of Tim we were beginning to believe in the other world, and life before and after death, in a continuum of existence that saw the spark of Divinity in each one walking the earth.

It was, however, a great sadness that Tim had written none of this down. It would have made such a difference to have a book written by him containing all the teachings. We remembered what we could, and often in conversation one of us would recall "Tim always said…" as if we were afraid of forgetting. Then one day, years later, in high summer, an American friend called Jean Sayre-Adams came to stay, bringing with her as a thank you gift *Emmanuel's Book - a Manual for Living Comfortably in the Cosmos*.[17] The book was written by Pat Rodegast and was a compilation of messages from the spirit guide Emmanuel. It was published in 1997, long after Tim died, yet, as we opened the book and began to read, it was as if he were standing there speaking to us. As well as his voice in my head, I now had a book in my hands. My joy and relief knew no bounds. The language was Tim's language and the teaching echoed everything that he had said. It was a perfect gift and I still have that original copy, endlessly thumbed and falling to pieces, in spite of many strips of Sellotape.

Chapter 9
Love and Death

By now, we were spreading our work far and wide through a network of support groups around the country. I had given up my work with BBC radio in order to concentrate on the charity, but I still heard occasional references to documentaries that I had made in the past decade. Relevant to Emmanuel's message of hope was a series I made with a psychic and clairvoyant called Tom Corbett. He was a gift to any producer: very amusing and articulate, with a fabulous Scottish accent, he helped me make a programme called *The Stately Ghosts of England*. He visited a number of stately homes full of history and ghosts. His stories were very entertaining and it was comforting to hear how he was able to release the poor, benighted souls and send them into the Light. "So you have no doubt at all that life goes on after death?" I asked him. "None at all," he responded heartily, and he went on to describe something that happened to him recently.

Tom had been involved in a car crash and although he only suffered bruises and scratches, the hospital decided to keep him in for the night. "I couldn't sleep after what had happened, and in the middle of the night I saw a procession coming down the corridor outside the women's ward opposite." I interrupted him to ask if he meant a real procession or something more 'other worldly'. "From the other world," he told me, "but of course they are as real to me as you are. They were laughing and jostling each other into the women's ward, and half way down on the left hand side they gathered right round the bed of a very old lady and very tenderly and lovingly they lifted her out of her body. She was immediately active and well, and clearly absolutely overjoyed. They were all embracing her, and exclaiming joyfully, and then at last the procession reformed with the lady at the head, and out of the ward they went, along the corridor and off."

Tom said the sight of all this filled him with great joy and he dozed till morning. When the morning staff came on duty he asked the senior nurse to verify that there had been a death in the night in the women's ward. "Mr Corbett, we don't talk about death here!" she exploded. So Tom had to wait for a friendly cleaner to come to his cubicle, and she agreed to find out for him. She came back later with the information: the old lady was ninety-two and the time had been 2.15am. Tom had seen it all.

When that part of the radio programme was transmitted on air some weeks later, the telephone lines were jammed with callers, saying, "That was the most comforting thing I have ever heard. Why don't they say things like that in church? It would make us all really happy to know that death is like that."

More than once I had the thought that the key to understanding life and death lay in this direction. The puzzle was that often it was only people with psychic gifts that had anything to say that was helpful - most others, especially scientists and the religious, poured scorn on such ideas. They maintained there was no proof, that near-death experience research carried no weight, however impressive it was. The body is just closing down, they said, and these are the physical symptoms. It was such a pity. Why, I wondered, was it so difficult to believe in these stories when the faith and religion that we had inherited was also pretty incredible? The Bible is the Word of God they said; yes, but written by men, inspired though they may have been. Thousands of years of culture have reinforced the message of the Bible, yet there is no inclusion of information we most need when facing the end of life. Eternal life is a mystery, they say. We just have to wait and see, and hope for the best.

So it was with great interest that I read Dr Raymond Moody's book *Glimpses of Eternity – An Investigation into Shared Death Experiences*[18] that tells about relatives sitting with the dying who left their bodies and accompanied the deceased on the first part of the journey into the next life. A medical colleague of Dr Moody, Dr Jamieson, told her story. She was visiting her mother when she went in to cardiac arrest. Greatly shocked, Dr Jamieson went to resuscitate her when she said she felt herself lift up out of her body - she was looking down at her own body and that of her now-deceased mother. "Being out-of-body took me aback," she said, "as I was trying to get my bearings I suddenly became aware that my mother was now hovering with me in spirit form." As she calmly said farewell to her mother, who was smiling and happy, Dr Jamieson saw something else. "I looked in the corner of the room and became aware of a breach in the universe that was pouring light like water coming from a broken pipe. Out of that light came people I had known for years, deceased friends of my mother." As Dr Jamieson watched, her mother drifted off into the light. The last Dr Jamieson saw of her mother, she said, she was having a very tender reunion with all of her friends. "Then the tube closed down in an almost spiral fashion and the light was gone," she said. She found herself back in her body, standing next to her deceased mother, totally puzzled about what had just happened.

Others have had the same experience and it has helped them erase some of their fears around dying and convinced them that life goes on. Elizabeth Kubler-Ross often commented how strange it was that people who had literally been to death's door in an out-of-body experience returned full of hope and joy. Their brush with death did not leave them depressed – quite the opposite. They became optimistic and determined to make the very best of the life that remained to them. It was a very real turning point in their lives and they saw dying as something they would no longer dread.

It is a pity that all this is shrouded in mystery and is not made common knowledge. What a difference it would make to us all to learn such things at our mother's knee. We would then see the journey of life in a quite different way. I suppose that in times past, our spiritual elders and betters wanted to keep us anxious in order to make us conform and toe the line. The sad thing is that if humanity had been reassured about the end of physical life and the immediate transit into the spiritual realm, people would have been happy and optimistic. Such people behave well and don't need controlling. Anxiety and fear breed negativity, and lead to all the difficulties of life that we know so well.

This concern about our final destiny is as old as the hills. Socrates said that the most important thing in life is understanding the immortality of the soul. Einstein at the end of his astonishingly creative time on earth said that the really important question was: "Does the source of life love me?" Knowing that we are loved makes all the difference and final words are often all about love. This was most evident as the twin towers were collapsing on 9/11. Scrambling to get out of the doomed building everyone shouted words of love into their mobile phones. We are concerned day by day with many things, but when the chips are truly down, there is only love and love is the one thing that endures.

Love is all that exists.

Love is the universal communication,
It is the energy that has created the
Universe and is keeping it going.
God is love.
All matter is formed by love.
There is an organic love
That speaks to everyone
If only they could but hear.
A leaf holds together
For love.

Love can turn the world around
And it does.
What did you think was spinning your planet
If it wasn't love?
And what do you think the fires of your sun consist of
And the cells of your body
And the stars in your sky
And the consciousness in your heart?
It is all love.

Emmanuel[19]

Chapter 10
Dark Clouds Gather

Our precious Centre in Clifton Village in Bristol was suffused with love. Our bid to purchase this former nunnery had been favoured by the Mother Superior who believed so strongly in the work we were doing. People coming in through the beautiful Georgian entrance with its curved and perfectly proportioned fanlight above the great oak door always spoke of their first impression of coming to us in their hour of need. They said it was as if some wonderful warm blanket was wrapped around them from their first moment with us. Celia said that there was a great angelic presence in the spacious entrance hall. She said it had the energy of the Holy Mother and it lovingly greeted each one as they entered. Not for the first time I wished I could see in this way too. It would have been so wonderful to have a glimpse of this other world that surrounded us, but I couldn't, although it was something I could feel intuitively, as could many of my colleagues.

It was because we all worked within this atmosphere of love and healing that it never occurred to us that anyone might wish us harm. It was absolutely obvious that we were doing only good. In our day to day work, we welcomed all visitors and never suspected their motives. However, for some years our experience had begun to change, at least in our engagement with the wider world, through the media. One day, before the move to Grove House, a television researcher had visited us from Glasgow asking if his company could make a film about us. We said they were welcome to visit but that while we were still in the early stages of our work we were not keen to commit to film. We felt we were doing a pilot study to begin with, and then we became so busy we didn't think TV exposure was a good idea. Understanding this, the young man nevertheless journeyed all the way to Bristol to have a day with us.

He was not allowed to join clients in their private sessions with the doctor, healer or counsellor, but remained in the group that spent most of the morning with Penny. It was nearly lunchtime and I was in the kitchen laying the large family table for the coming meal when this young man came out of Penny's group and made his way to where I was. I was surprised to see him and soon noticed that he was very upset. He was almost in tears. I sat him down, thinking that hearing people telling their stories was upsetting him. "No," he said, "it's not that. They are amazing and Penny is just wonderful with them. I am tremendously touched by everything I have heard and seen since I got here this morning. But I feel I have to tell you that I came here under false pretences. My boss had heard about your work. He makes programmes exposing fraudulent companies and organisations." He told me the name of his boss and the title of the programme, which of course I recognised. "But," he said, his voice quivering, "You are not like that at all. We had the idea you were milking money out of these people, and you are actually not charging them at all." "We only charge a pound for their lunch," I interrupted. "We thought you were steering them away from hospital treatments with false claims for quack therapies, but you're not. I feel so ashamed and I think I should leave now."

I demurred and told him lunch was nearly ready. "What I would really like to do is to come and do a proper study with you all here. That would be wonderful. The story is a tremendous one and I am going to see if I can convert my boss." It was lucky that at that moment everyone came down the stairs for lunch and our conversation ended. I had certainly made up my mind that in no way would we consider embarking on something that could become dangerous to us if it got out of control. I thought it was a pity that such a genuine and likeable person was working in such a negative field and I wished him well when his taxi came for him at the end of the afternoon.

When everyone had gone, I shared the story with the others who all agreed we had had a lucky escape. It was, however, strange that soon after this we were contacted by BBC producers of the *40 Minutes* series asking if they could come and see us. Being more aware of our vulnerability we stipulated that they must spend three days observing what we were doing before we would consider their request to make a programme about us. Astonishingly they agreed and Roger Mills and Annie Paul came to see us for the required time. They became very enthusiastic about making a film and we spent long hours with them making sure they understood what we were doing, and checking whether there was an ulterior motive. We all liked them a great deal and began to feel that here at last were media people we could trust.

The plan was for them to make one programme but when they began to look into the whole process of filming they thought the best plan was to follow one set of new clients through their time with us. We had no knowledge of who these clients might be, because we hadn't met them. They were enrolled by the BBC and filming began in their homes before they came, and on the train or in the car as they made their way to Bristol. Penny was on the doorstep greeting their arrival and we progressed through our usual programme, hardly conscious of the cameraman and Annie Paul who managed to fade in to the background in an extraordinary way. We all soon relaxed and got on with what we were doing.

Back in their studio they realised that it was impossible to make only one programme, and in the end there were five. The quality of the filming was extraordinarily good and we were involved all the time. The camera crew became very popular with us all. Penny treated the cameraman for his addiction to smoking with acupuncture needles in his ears, and when they were filming clients at home they offered to mow the lawn and clean the windows. It was hard to think of life without them.

Annie Paul was particularly sensitive when filming Leonora from Cornwall. We could see when she arrived on the first day that she was near the end of her life. She was radiantly beautiful, intelligent and engaging and had a wonderful presence. She knew she was dying but wanted what she called 'a summer for the children'. She took to every part of our therapeutic programme wholeheartedly and as she improved her nutrition and worked with meditation and visualisation at home, a bit of vigour and strength returned. Annie filmed her walking the beautiful Cornish coastal paths with her family and there was no doubting the joy and delight on her face as she spoke to the camera.

However there came a time when she was mostly in bed and she continued to speak to the camera. "As my body is flowing away from me," she said, "my spirit is rising. I have all I need. My doctor is keeping me comfortable and my healer comes every day." She indicated the pile of books on her bed, all spiritual titles. In the final programme, after Leonora's death, Annie asked Leonora's husband if the end had been like that. He watched the footage of Leonora on a monitor, tears moving down his cheeks, and he nodded. "It was absolutely wonderful," he said of her last moments.

On March 17, 1983, on the afternoon of the transmission of the first programme of the series (which they had called *A Gentle Way With Cancer*), I received a phone call from the Bristol Evening Post asking for my reaction to the fact that the BBC was having to cancel showing it that evening. This was the first we had heard of it, and I was shocked and dismayed. Why should such a thing happen?

The phone went again and it was Roger Mills, who was in overall charge of the programme. He said not to worry and that they had managed to persuade the powers that be to let this one through. But why I asked should they want to cancel it anyway? Roger explained that there had been a review of the film in the Sunday press and a number of high up medical people had leaned on BBC management to stop transmission. "We told them that it would be an even bigger story if this got out because the programme was cancelled, so they agreed to let it through. But I don't know about the following films." In the event all the films, each one a wonderful human story, were shown, though the programme makers were forced to add a question mark at the end of the title *A Gentle Way With Cancer?* The BBC management also insisted that a sixth programme was added: a discussion with three medical practitioners.

During that year the subject of research came up and meetings were held with medical professionals. Finally, in September 1984, Dr Clair Chilvers and statistician Dr Douglas Easton, both from the Institute of Cancer Research, drafted a proposal for research on the survival of patients attending the Centre. Funding for the five-year Survival of Patients study was approved in 1986 by the Imperial Cancer Research Fund and the Cancer Research Campaign.

The plan was for 334 of our breast cancer clients to be matched with 461 patients from three NHS hospitals and followed for five years to make it clear whether the Bristol Programme had anything to recommend it. We saw no reason why this should not proceed. We were absolutely confident that people were benefiting from our programme. Taking our work into a wider field made a lot of sense and being underpinned by reputable research was just what we needed. It was the one piece of our jigsaw that was missing and we looked forward to completing the circle. In the event the circle became a noose around our necks that almost took the life from us.

Chapter 11
A Sense of Connection

The Bristol Cancer Help Centre had started life as a pilot project following Penny's experience at Issel's clinic in Germany and our meeting with Dr Alec Forbes. We forgot the temporary nature of our endeavour, however, as month succeeded month and we became deeply engaged with what we were doing. We were delighted how much benefit clients gained from learning about healthy nutrition, having healing sessions or counselling, or reading new material. We began to notice some clients who became seriously engaged with all aspects of the programme moved into a transformational state that changed everything about them. They described this new state as an awakening, and often spoke of their life before cancer as a sort of 'sleep walk'.

In the cancer world, people spoke of 'fighting spirit' as being the significant factor that influenced the outcome of the disease, and certainly it seemed clear that being hopeless and helpless had a powerful negative effect; but we began to think we were seeing something of very great significance. Some seemed to move to a deeper state of being that enabled them to stand up to their illness with fire in the soul. They spoke of feeling close to God, of experiencing angelic power, of losing all fear, and of knowing that life went on after death.

Tim Tiley always used to remind us that the work we had put our hands to was spiritual work. He emphasised that every aspect of our work had a spiritual element and that we must keep this constantly in mind. The busier we became and the more our finances worried us, the more we needed his warning. And yet the extraordinary thing was that, worrying as things inevitably were, nevertheless all our needs were met, usually at the eleventh hour.

Bonds between members of our group strengthened. We felt so strongly connected to our clients and it seemed they were powerfully connected to each other, too. The relationships between those of us working together seemed to be shot through with a force field of energy.

My mother used to tell a story that we all loved. She had been widowed for several years before she felt able to venture abroad to stay with friends. Bob, an airline pilot, and Betty, her neighbours in Buckinghamshire, had an apartment overlooking the sea in Beirut and invited her to stay with them. It was an ideal holiday for such an unfamiliar traveller, and my mother travelled out on a plane piloted by Captain Bob. Days were spent exploring with Betty, while Bob took his great aircraft back to London. The two women spent happy evenings on the balcony overlooking the sea, chatting and sipping gin and tonic.

The only thing that my mother did not take to was the rather large aviary that occupied one corner of the balcony filled with exotic and squawking birds. It was almost impossible to speak over the din, and the only way to silence them was to place a heavy blanket over the cage. One evening, all was quiet as Betty and my mother watched the light gradually fade from the sky. Suddenly, in spite of the protective blanket, the birds arose as one to make a colossal din. "Good God, Bet!" my mother cried. "What's the matter with your wretched birds?" "Oh that must be Bob's plane up there," said Betty as she pointed to the sky out to sea. "The birds always know when Bob is flying in. He will call in half an hour to say how soon he will be home." My mother asked how the birds knew that it was Bob and not another pilot and Betty replied, "They do. They just do. They are Bob's birds you see."

In 1999 biologist Rupert Sheldrake articulated a theory about the existence of 'morphic fields' between humans and between humans and animals. He put his collected research material into a book *Dogs That Know When their Owners are Coming Home*[20], and said that telepathy (Greek for 'distant feeling') exists between humans and animals if they are closely bonded. He says that everything, from molecules and organisms to societies, and even entire galaxies, are shaped by morphic fields. These fields, he says, have a morphic resonance, a cumulative memory of similar systems through culture and time, so that species of animals and plants 'remember' not only how to look, but also how to act. He speaks of the self-organising properties of biological systems. "All morphic fields have an inherent memory given by morphic resonance and must interact with electromagnetic fields and quantum fields," he claims.

How this interaction occurs remains unclear but he continues to research the many strange and coincidental things that occur between humans and animals, humans and humans, and the bewildering and extraordinary synchronistic things that happen in our everyday lives. Perhaps the palpable energy that was flowing between us and between clients was a morphic field?

I was fortunate enough recently to have lunch with Rupert Sheldrake and some other like-minded friends. As I recounted my mother's Beirut adventure it opened a floodgate of similar stories. Morphic fields, we learned, were elastic - when flocks of birds wheel and loop in the sky, although many thousand, they act as of one mind and in an instant. The same applies to shoals of fish. Possibly it also accounts for instantaneous reactions in the human body, involving billions of cells. Information does not need to pass one by one, as might be imagined; it broadcasts itself in an instant.

Rupert said telepathy between humans depended on a close link of affection between bonded individuals. I remember when my daughter was at boarding school, she often used to call me mid-morning to ask for my prayers. One day she had a maths test after break and hadn't done the homework - only prayer could save the day! I had just made coffee for a friend and we sat at the table when the phone rang. I picked up the receiver and heard my daughter's voice loud and clear. "Hello Mummy," she said several times. I responded with my usual greeting and then asked if she had put in the right money and pressed the button to activate the phone. I could hear her but she evidently could not hear me. I relayed this to my friend who was sitting close by, before finally giving up and replacing the receiver. "She will try again in a moment," I said.

However, there were no more calls until that evening when my daughter's familiar greeting rang out loud and clear. This time she evidently could hear me. "Darling," I said, "I could hear you this morning when you called but you clearly couldn't hear me." There was a long pause. Then my daughter almost whispered, "Mummy. I wanted to call you but there was a queue for the phone and the bell went before I could have my turn. I didn't get to the phone." Now it was my turn to pause and think. "But I heard your voice," I said. "My phone rang and Anne was with me and she heard it too. She heard me speaking to you." In some way my daughter had spoken to me and, guessing she needed my prayers, I prayed. "I did well in the test," came the triumphant response.

Rupert Sheldrake went on to tell us how it might be possible in the long run to understand the mystery of communication with the Divine. "The core of all religion is mystical experience, expressed through the practices and cultures of social groups and communities," he said. "It is the common thread."

I was not the only one at that lunch table thinking that we live in a truly magical world. As I drove home I thought that the secret was to find a way to make the magic work for us in our everyday lives. I also saw with immense clarity that belief in a Higher Power is not an optional extra for people who like that sort of thing: it is as vital as any other thing that sustains life. Is the malaise and distress we see around us today in western culture with its addiction and depression perhaps an indication of what is missing? It is only in the last century that people have sloughed off the old faiths and religions and the beliefs, rituals and practices that go with them. Generations have now grown up with a gap where traditional faith and belief once resided.

Timothy Freke in his book *The Mystery Experience*[21] speaks of people waking up to a connectedness with a sense of astonishment and with the exclamation 'Wow!' on their lips. He says he has spent a lifetime exploring worldwide spiritual traditions because at their heart they all offer ways to awaken the 'Wow'. They are guides to transforming consciousness and opening to a love affair with life. He calls this passionate state 'enlivenment' when he is intensely present and in love with the moment, "then, my mundane life seems marvellous. The familiar world becomes a wonderland.

"The presence of God is a reality in my life but for me God isn't a great spirit that is separate from me. God is a primal oneness that is conscious through me." All our personal loves, he says, arise from this great love, the 'God Love' in us. It is a love so big it has no limits.

I think of the thousands of dear, wonderful people who have been our clients over so many years and wonder if the most important thing we did was to help them discover their personal 'Wow' factor. For some it may have been the healing effect of being surrounded by love and compassion; for others unlocking a spirituality; for others the relaxation and release sensed during massage. Their connectedness to each other and the bonds that grew between them, I am sure, played a part, too.

One of these dear clients wrote: "The peace and tranquillity experienced on entering the building was immeasurable. For one week I was free of the pressures of the outside world. I could concentrate on myself, absorb the calm and love, and think about my life. There was a quiet, vibrant atmosphere and no one looked at you with fear in their eyes. So began a week that was to change our lives."

The 'Wow' can lead to transformation, and this high-energy process affects the physical body. Often the love that wraps around the clients as they enter the building is the start of the process. Love is the great healer: it is compassion in action and it loosens the bonds of fear, allowing people to relax and be themselves. This is the 'safe place' of Penny's dreams. She always said how helpful it was to be bathed in an atmosphere of loving kindness to help the healing process to begin.

Chapter 12
The Storm Breaks

Tribulation broke about our heads in 1990 when the Imperial Cancer Research Fund told us a press conference was to be held at its headquarters on September 5th. The conference was held ahead of publication of their research study in *The Lancet* three days later. We had almost forgotten that this research programme was rumbling on month by month. Our clients were recruited into it and responded positively and in depth to the questionnaires that were sent them regularly, but members of staff were not involved.

We discovered hundreds of journalists had been invited to the press conference and Penny and Dr Wetzler, our senior doctor at the time, decided to agree to sit on the platform in front of the press.

Immediately afterwards, Penny called me from London but I couldn't hear what she was saying - it was distorted by her extreme distress. She was in a phone box near Lincoln's Inn Fields and all I could hear was sobbing. When at last she managed to find her voice she said how the enormous crowd of reporters, television cameras and radio crews already had the press release. All too late it had come into Penny's hands. It gave notice of the shocking results of the interim two-year study. The research had found that women who followed the Bristol programme, as well as having orthodox treatment, were nearly three times more likely to relapse and nearly twice as likely to die as the control patients who only received hospital treatment.[22]

Once I heard and understood what Penny was saying I could well understand her tears. We had given our lives to this work. We knew that people were benefiting and often outliving their prognosis. These findings simply could not be right and as Penny had told reporters at the time: "There has to be a ghost in the machine. It can't make sense that the therapies we are conducting could be harmful."

But what were we to do? I went to find Christopher and poured out the terrible news. He held me close to him and said that what we were doing was good, and of God, and in the end something good would come of it. At the time it was hard to see. We were entering our own crisis nightmare that obliterated the sun and plunged us into blackness.

The press and media had a field day. It was just a few days before the actual publishing of *The Lancet*, so they had no means of studying the actual document. They latched on to the fact that Prince Charles had opened our Centre in 1983 and that he was closely associated with us. This made the story irresistible and news about our downfall was splashed on the front pages. It was the leading news item that night and discussion followed on and on. It could not have been worse.

Penny did her best for us, fighting our corner in televised discussions and radio talk shows, but she had no idea of what had gone wrong, or how these results had come to be. She returned from these gruelling events pale and exhausted. She was pouring out her last drop of energy for her beloved Centre and was losing ground. Looking back years later, I dated the return and spread of her cancer to this terrible time.

But worse was happening for our clients. Families were exposed to all the hype about the damaging effect of the Bristol programme. Children were immediately upset and concerned for parents who had been to Bristol. "I woke in the middle of the night," one of our clients told us "to find my twelve-year-old daughter standing at the bottom of my bed. I asked her what she wanted and she told me she was worried I might die in the night and was checking if I was still breathing." Our worry and distress turned to anger. How dared these people do so much damage, so needlessly and thoughtlessly? We needed to fight back, but in all honesty, we didn't know how.

Our four-month waiting list vanished overnight. Our fundraising adventures dried up equally fast. 'No smoke without fire' was a catchword for people with money to give. If these people had put on a piece of research in order to destroy us, they couldn't have done better. It looked as if we were finished.

We tried to get some of the data from the cancer charities to go through it and try to understand what had gone wrong, but our request was refused. One of our doctors, who had been trained in research studies in the past, pored over *The Lancet* article and suggested that the point of recruitment was probably the problem. And so it proved to be: our clients were entered into the study from the day they arrived to stay with us at Bristol. That might have been a number of years on from first diagnosis, and into secondary spread. The control clients were from the NHS Cancer Registry which entered them at diagnosis. Apples were being compared with pears. By the end of the year a correction was put in *The Lancet* by the Institute of Cancer Research, but there was no press conference and hardly any publicity. The original study has never been removed from the literature.

Our clients who had taken part in the study were upset and angry. They had been filling in endless forms as part of the research programme. They had added long descriptions of the transformation they were experiencing that affected every part of their lives. They spoke of the changes they were making in lifestyle and purpose. Filling in these forms at regular intervals was a big thing for them and they thought everything counted in the research protocol. Little did they know that their 'controls' were just names plucked from a registry: not actual participants who were also writing essays about their experiences.

So distressed were they that they formed a group called the Bristol Survey Support Group, with two dynamic women at the helm: Heather Goodare and Isla Bourke. The group met regularly to try to see what could be done to repair the damage. They felt let down by us at Bristol because we didn't come out fighting. They told us that we had taught them to fight for their lives, and now we, the teachers, were sinking under the strain of our own disempowerment. It was true.

We took legal advice, which was very expensive. In January 1994, the Charity Commission issued a press release saying a formal inquiry found "procedures for the supervision of research were insufficient to ensure that charity funds granted to independent researchers were properly controlled. The charities also lent their names to the publication of the research without ensuring that it was soundly based." Even the Cancer Research Campaign said that the researchers made "an honest scientific mistake".

Despite this we did not pursue a legal route. One cancer charity suing another cancer charity would be an unedifying sight. We consulted PR people and they were also at a loss, and almost as expensive. Money was running out and we had hardly any clients. We had to make staff redundant and return to the few of us who had always worked for nothing. One of our most junior doctors, Rosy Daniel, who cared passionately for the Centre, offered to work unpaid if she could manage to merge working for us into her GP programme. So that was how we looked into the future, praying that this time of trial would pass, and that we could begin again. Someone said this was our organisation's cancer experience; we certainly began to understand more about the power of crisis to change our lives.

The Bristol Survey Support Group met regularly, sometimes coming to Bristol and often in London. They were tremendously feisty and courageous in approaching people for help. In a way they were in a better position to seek favours than we were. They were cancer patients and they were seeking redress. Finally they made a television programme with Channel 4, *Cancer Positive*. In it they managed to get apologies from Sir Walter Bodmer of the Imperial Cancer Research Fund and Professor Gordon McVie of Cancer Research Campaign. It was a triumph. They sent a video of it to Prince Charles who immediately came back asking how he could help. It seemed that we had turned a corner and Rosy Daniel devised a new programme for us that contained all the essential ingredients of therapy, but was much less expensive to run.

Little by little we began again. Christopher always said something good would come out of the crisis, and it was this: we had survived the crisis period all working for nothing and we lived in an atmosphere of prayer and faith. We would light candles and sit in a circle holding hands, asking for the help we needed. Help came in many and astonishing ways, and bit by bit we became busy once again.

The whole time of crisis had taken a great deal out of Penny. She began to complain of backache and thought she must have a trapped nerve. She put up with it for some time and finally had a scan to see what the trouble was. The cancer had spread to the spine. The stress of the last years had taken its toll. It was devastating. Surgery followed and radiotherapy. We had to learn how to work without her at the Centre while she moved through a great deal of rehabilitation to get her strength back. Rosy had brought Jane Sen, a most amazing cook, to work at the Centre; now we were eating gourmet food at every meal, and Jane packaged up goodie bags for Penny at home or in hospital, so that she had all she needed.

She was surrounded by love from us all as well as at home, and just a few months later she organised a cycling holiday in Brittany for the family. She returned to us renewed and able to take up a certain amount of work. We were really busy once again and the crisis began to seem like a thing of the past.

Chapter 13
Preparing for Death

Penny looked really well when she returned from her holiday in France and so it was devastating to me when I learned from a medical friend that she was now receiving palliative care. At the time this was a fairly new concept and one that was growing with the hospice movement. In no way did I associate palliative care with someone who looked as well as Penny did. My consultant friend went on to say she had great powers of recovery and would no doubt put up a good fight, but with the cancer spreading in her body the original picture had changed. I kept this conversation to myself, not wanting to upset my colleagues, but in my own mind I began to question at what point in the life cycle should we move from a determined fight to get well, to preparation for death. After all, unless we die in an accident suddenly and without warning, we are all going to face the beginning of the end. What do we say to ourselves when the scenery changes and we are looking at the final curtain?

The more I thought about it, the more it seemed to me that for all our work and spiritual practice, we are all unprepared. It is extraordinary that when with our intellects we absolutely know that every life ends in death, nevertheless we act as if, and presume, that we are going on forever! It is a strange trick of human optimism. And then, suddenly, we have to face the truth. We are forced to think about what part of us survives and what sort of life awaits us beyond the grave if, that is, we trust in any sort of survival. Whatever our beliefs, there clearly is work to be done, and it is wise to do it while we still have life and limb. The work starts with the questions "who am I?", "for what purpose have I come into this lifetime?" and considers "where am I going?" and "will I remain in touch with those I love?"

Penny again let go of much of her routine work at the Centre and concentrated on the second part of her autobiography. The first part, *Gentle Giants*[23], had been published to great acclaim. I often popped over to see her and enjoyed her beautiful watercolour paintings, her craft work, crochet and knitting. David had set up his own business by this time, working out of outbuildings at home. He was able to get on with work and yet be on hand to see to Penny's needs.

"He is an absolute angel," Penny said to me one afternoon over the teacups. "Nothing is too much trouble. I don't know how I would manage without him." As her physical difficulties multiplied, their love grew deeper. She refilled my teacup, holding one arm around the beautiful silver haired cat that was sleeping in her lap. "Sometimes," she went on slowly, searching for words, "sometimes I wonder if I should just let go. The way things are, David is completely tied to my side. Obviously it will take him a year or so to get over losing me, but then he has his life ahead of him to get on with living."

I was silent for a long time. Then I looked at her and asked, "How does that make you feel?" Tears streamed down her cheeks. "I shall be so sorry to leave him, and the children. It will be so hard to part with this lovely house and the garden…" She waved her hand towards the late roses glowing in the early evening sun. She held the cat more closely to her. She began speaking of each of her three children. They were all now in their late twenties, living away from home, running successful lives. "They are all doing well but I think they can't quite move on because of me. It might be better for them …" A long silence followed. Then she brightened a little. "It would be such a relief not to keep fighting;

108

just gently letting things take their course."

I drove home with a heavy heart, wondering whether it might be that we can influence our departure once we are clear that we are ready to go. I spent some time that evening talking to Christopher, asking him if we had power to influence how and when we depart. "Usually the power we have is at the deep level of the soul, and we are not actually conscious of it," he said. "I have seen many people in residential homes who ask over and over, 'Why doesn't the Lord come for me?' They seem unable to die when they want to. They live on and on."

Christopher went on to remind me of a story that our friend the Reverend Gordon Barker had told us some years before. Gordon was assisting a catholic priest called Father Andrew in running a weekend workshop at Hawkwood College in Gloucestershire. It was something that he had done a number of times and they were always magical occasions because Father Andrew was a mystic and had access through his psychic gifts to information about the other world. We never met him but gathered that his teaching was very similar to Tim's.

Gordon told us that after supper with the participants on the Friday evening, Father Andrew outlined the shape of the course that he would be teaching, and then proceeded with a short service of prayer and blessing, before sending everyone off to bed. Gordon and Andrew had rooms in the old part of the house and they enjoyed a hot drink and a quiet chat. Suddenly, though, everything changed. "Gordon, my dear friend, would you mind if I died tonight?" Gordon said he almost dropped his mug of coffee. "Died?" he stammered, "What do you mean, died?" Andrew, though elderly, looked perfectly well. It didn't seem possible. Was this some joke? But it clearly wasn't. "It is time I went and this is a good time to go, but if it is too much for you..." Gordon was now taking it in. Andrew was obviously not talking about suicide - such a thing would never enter his head - but he clearly meant what he was saying. Somehow he was planning to leave his body forthwith,

with the result that the workshop would have to be cancelled. All those dear people were expecting wonderful teaching, and they would be overwhelmingly disappointed.

Gordon drew breath and asked, "What about the workshop?" "That is no problem - you will do it!" Now Gordon really spluttered, saying he was incapable of teaching Andrew's course. "You won't have to," he was told. "I will be there at your side. You will just speak the words that I give you." For a moment Gordon thought he was going mad but Andrew was in earnest. "You will have no worries. The words will come."

At last they parted and Gordon prepared himself for sleep, but remained wide-eyed throughout the night. Several times he got out of bed to go to Andrew's room to see if he was all right and then paused at the door and returned to bed. At last dawn brought light to the room and he got up. Andrew's door was shut and all was silent. Releasing the catch Gordon gently pushed open the door, and found Andrew neatly lying in his bed. He was gone.

The household was greatly distressed when informed of the news, and Gordon put on his priest's robes and led a service of commemoration and dedication. Then he offered an hour's break and said he would begin the teaching after coffee. When all were finally assembled Gordon faced the crowded lecture hall and calmed himself with a few deep breaths. It was then that he realised Andrew was at his side. He could feel his presence clearly and hear his voice. "This is much better than being in my tight black suit," said Andrew. "On we go." Sentence followed sentence, with Gordon speaking to the audience, who all settled quietly with pen and notebook ready. Time flowed on and the first session was complete when the gong went for lunch. Andrew had been as good as his word. The teaching was his.

Gordon told us that he managed the whole weekend successfully and people said as they left, "It could have been Father Andrew speaking! Thank you, Gordon." If only they'd known. Christopher and I talked over Gordon's story again and again, and

Christopher reminded me that Jesus himself had said, "I will not leave you comfortless: I will come to you." It is possible that we are not left bereaved and entirely alone if we can quieten ourselves sufficiently to tune in to that other dimension.

Chapter 14
Going Home

Penny died on February 3, 1999, exactly six months after our conversation over tea. It was twenty years since her first diagnosis of cancer. Snowdrops were coming up in my garden but, welcome as they were, it seemed a very long and bitter winter. At the funeral and the memorial service that followed, Penny's younger daughter spoke words from Penny's favourite poem, *The North Ship*, by Philip Larkin[24]:

If I can keep against all argument
Such image of a snow-white unicorn.
Then, as I pray, it may for sanctuary
Descend at last to me,
And put into my hand its golden horn.

The world seemed a lot emptier. Penny had been such a presence and had inspired so many. Clients had identified with her and her death took away some of their confidence. I felt sad for a long time and filled my time with work and speaking engagements. One evening I was with a group speaking about our work when an elderly lady told me that Penny was standing at my side. She gave an extraordinarily detailed and accurate account of her appearance, what she was like and many details of her personality. "What could be more natural than that she should continue to help you?" the lady went on. "Wouldn't you do the same in her place?" I couldn't but agree. As I drove the many miles back home that night I felt as if some gift had been put into my hand, and I was immensely cheered.

The more that I think about the extraordinary blessing of the life that I shared with Christopher and the friendships we shared with Penny and Tim, the more it seems that we together were on a quest for meaning. The teaching that we received from Tim moved us on the path: it led to the healing ministry, from which grew the Bristol Cancer Help Centre. Our work there was far more profound than teaching good lifestyle skills. It was a process leading to transformation.

Had we but known it, it was all about what Danah Zohar calls Spiritual Intelligence – "an ability to be guided by the soul, to live a life at a deeper level of meaning." Danah describes Spiritual Intelligence[25] as another part of ourselves that can be developed and enhanced. It is not about religion, rather it is the part of ourselves that seeks to find meaning and goodness both in our own actions and the world around us and we can use it to solve questions of importance to our souls. I realised as I read her marvellous book that Spiritual Intelligence is for me the unifying lynch pin of our holistic approach at the Centre. Danah Zohar says, describing Spiritual Intelligence, or SQ: "Like Intellectual Intelligence (IQ) and Emotional Intelligence (EQ), it makes up our ultimate and fully developed awareness, enabling us to ask fundamental and ultimate questions to satisfy our longing for meaning in our lives."

She feels that a life of religious study and belief does not necessarily confer a high level of Spiritual Intelligence, nor does it preclude it. For myself, as I read Danah Zohar's words, it was as if I had suddenly found a more scientific language with which to explain the hitherto more mystical path of my own soul journey and purpose. I have always been fascinated by scientific exploration into the functioning of the brain – here was a book that explores the neural connectivity in the brain specifically as it relates or 'vibrates' to meditative or spiritual practices.

On my own journey I had found huge release from the rigid interpretation of the Bible I had received in childhood through Christopher's own understanding and study. His years of exploration begun at theological college continued throughout his life, his deep knowledge of the history of the Church illuminating many hours of discussion between us.

Danah Zohar holds this perspective on conventional religious structure:

> *Conventional religion is an externally imposed set of rules and beliefs. It is top down, inherited from priests and prophets and holy books, or absorbed through the family and tradition. SQ is internal, a facility that allows the brain to find and use meaning in the solution of problems. It can guide us from within because it is the soul's intelligence. Healing and wisdom come from this part of our being and from it comes our desire for religion.*

Had we helped people gain new perspective and vision as they moved through the cancer crisis? Certainly we tried to help them make some sense of their experience. Many clients have said to us over the years, "Nothing less than cancer would have woken me up. I was sleepwalking." If, with newly SQ-minted eyes, we can see crisis as a message sent in good faith from some higher part of our being - our soul perhaps - then we immediately lose that unpleasant concept that this unfortunate happening has been delivered as a judgement upon us from some vengeful deity.

No wonder Tim had kept repeating: "Remember, your work at the Centre is spiritual work." As we took on more and more staff it was a struggle to keep the message clear. Even more of a problem was the confusion between Spiritual Intelligence and religion. Not having Danah Zohar's work to hand at the time, articulating the message was not easy. It so often became mixed up with religion and as we moved into the new millennium more and more people began to abandon any religious attachment. What we were looking for was an everyday holiness, a homespun self-reflectiveness, a desire to change to a higher way of being and sacredness of meaning, living from the deepest centre of the self. Not for the first time I wished that Tim was still with us.

As things unfolded in the year 2000, that yearning increased exponentially: at the beginning of May, Christopher had a heart attack. Life-changing crisis had come home to roost. He was seventy-six.

As a family we had completely escaped illness, hospital and health worries; we had coughs and colds, the occasional bronchitis, but nothing serious, no broken bones. My three babies were all born at home with a minimum of intervention. Now suddenly here we were faced with the sort of thing that we thought only happened to other people. We were away from home, having spent the night in a hotel in Plymouth where I was giving a lecture. Christopher was free and went out to explore the town when he began to experience the sort of pain that makes you hail a taxi to the nearest hospital.

I came out of the lecture hall to find someone waiting for me with a note in her hand. I was to ring Derriford Hospital. Greatly concerned, I found a public phone and called. "Your husband has had a heart attack. Please come immediately," I was told. He had been perfectly well at breakfast: what could have occurred to bring this on? I rushed to his side and found a very crowded emergency ward with hardly room to stand between the beds. "I am so sorry, my darling, but I am afraid I am having a heart attack," said Christopher. His face was flushed but he was completely calm. I alerted the children and in no time they were Plymouth-bound on a train. The crowded ward became even more densely packed as we clustered around the bed. Angioplasty removed the blockage but it was a number of days before we were allowed to take him home. Life had suddenly changed and we all realised that he had had a narrow escape.

For the first time I faced the thought that Christopher was as vulnerable as anyone else. I might lose him. Our work had always been with people living on the edge, people who faced this concept daily, and yet it was always a bit removed from us. Try as I would, I could not take in this new situation.

Christopher had been passed into the care of a wonderful cardiologist in Bristol and continued to have regular appointments with him. The consultant told us that before taking up cardiology, he had specialised in neurological disorders and those still interested him greatly. He watched the way Christopher walked into his room, the way several of his fingers twitched and shook from time to time, and at our second meeting he said to Christopher, "How long have you had Parkinson's disease?" We looked at him blankly. "Has Parkinson's been diagnosed?" he asked.

Heart attack, Parkinson's disease: our world was unravelling before our eyes. All those certainties by which we had lived suddenly toppled over. The healer who helped so many others was in trouble himself. Assisted by our children, we moved house to live in an easier sort of way and we adapted to a different, simpler lifestyle. And things were still good. I spent hours in the kitchen making fresh juices, wholesome soups and delicious meals to make the most of the health that Christopher still had.

The journey with Parkinson's held many frustrations for Christopher and occasionally my own frustration would spill over. I remember while I was busy cooking he would hover, unable to move, somewhere between the stove and the sink. He was anxious to help me, but I would want him out of my way. At the time I was studying Caroline Myss's book *Sacred Contracts*[26]. It was at the moment when impatience was about to boil over into exasperation that it came to me: this trial is here in my life to help me to practise patience. How can I learn to be patient without practice? So together we practised patience, faith, hope, trust, humility, courage and endurance. And love, of course, especially love.

Christopher became compliant and accepting: taking the pills and the vitamins, swallowing the juices and never complaining. Indeed, his loving affection grew towards me daily and I thought I could detect a new soul strength arising as his physical strength withdrew.

Of course we had many friends who were healers and on one bright, sunny Friday morning two of them came to give Christopher healing, and stayed on to have lunch with us. The healing ended and I started to prepare lunch for us all. Christopher moved towards where we were sitting and addressed me: "I love you, my darling, and I love our life together, but I want to go home." For a few moments I tried to take in what he was saying, realising its deeper meaning, before replying from a deep place within myself: "And I love you, my darling, and I also love our life together, but if you want to go home you must do so whenever you want to, and I will get on as best I can."

Our healer friends were there, holding us in prayer. They knew the power and depth of this exchange. Perhaps it was their healing energy that made the interaction possible. There was a long silence and I escaped over to the kitchen range. Conversation resumed as if nothing had happened, but it had and it was earth shattering.

There were practical things to be done: Living Wills to write, Powers of Attorney to sign. We were clearing the decks to be ready for what lay ahead. It began with night nurses, to give me a chance to sleep. Then the agency provided round the clock cover, and wonderful equipment came from the NHS to help us look after Christopher at home. This could have been a terrible time with the house so full of people, so many to feed and all privacy gone; but it wasn't. It was wonderful. The nurses all adored Christopher who flirted with them and encouraged them to tell him stories of home.

Most of our nurses were African and their stories were often of the terrible effects of AIDS on their families. Their sisters had died of it and the children were being cared for by the grannies while our nurses were earning the money to keep them all going. Most were Christian and when Christopher had been carefully tucked into bed at night, we all knelt around him, arms enfolded, to pray together. They prayed for us and we prayed for them. It was a powerful experience of the power of religion used at the highest level. The extraordinary thing was that, although Christopher had lost all his short-term memory, and often seemed very confused, nevertheless in these moments of prayer each evening he could recite long passages of liturgy from the services that he had conducted long years ago. And when he concluded with the Blessing there was no doubt that the priest was still with us.

Finally in 2006 it was clear that we could no longer manage at home. I found a place for him in a wonderful nursing home in Bristol. I sat with him one afternoon preparing to tell him of the arrangements I was making. I had rehearsed a little speech to explain that we could no longer continue as we were. I put my arm round him and began, only getting a little way into what I wanted to say. I was overwhelmed with grief and sobbed helplessly. I felt I was betraying him: turning him out. And suddenly the wonderful old Christopher was there comforting me. "It will be interesting to meet all those people. It will be like being in the outer courts of heaven," he said cheerily. I could not believe my ears.

With enormous courage he took an active part in deciding what furniture to take with him, which of the precious photos and mementos that reminded him of home. Once in the nursing home he made friends with all the staff and his room often rocked to laughter and music. A dear friend spent most mornings with him, arriving early to help with his breakfast, and I got there straight after lunch to be with him until bedtime. It was strange suddenly to have nothing to do - we had both always been so busy. I was enrolled in a campaign to knit squares for blankets, and over the year lost count of how many hundreds flew from my knitting needles.

The nursing home had a large and enchanting garden and unless it was raining we wrapped up and took ourselves there, Christopher in his large and comfortable wheelchair with me pushing as if my life depended on it. After a while I would need a rest and, finding one of the many convenient seats that graced the garden, we put Christopher's chair at an angle so that we were able to sit and hold hands. How many times in our over-busy life had we grumbled and said, "All I want to do is to sit in the sun and hold hands!" And there, because dementia had taken all short-term memory, we rehearsed services from the Prayer Book and enchanted each other with cadences of poetry. The brain, which had played so many cruel tricks on this dear and enlightened man, still held pockets of long remembered, precious words.

He was in the nursing home for exactly a year, and died in October 2007, six days before his eighty-fourth birthday. We were together for fifty-four years.

Chapter 15
The Move to Ham Green House

We didn't see the heart attack coming; we didn't realise Parkinson's disease was setting in. In the same way we didn't realise that something extraordinary was happening within our Centre when, along with many other clients suffering from cancer, a smart and beguiling girl called Nina Barough walked through the door. She had breast cancer and was in need of the help we could give. She received the tender, loving and skilled care for which we had become known. She knew a lot about health and fitness, and she told us about the power-walking that she had taken up with a number of her friends. Extraordinarily gifted in organisation and in inspiring people to join her, she was busy fundraising for cancer charities. Her health so greatly improved that she generously wanted to include us in her fundraising. Nina devised the MoonWalk, a marathon power-walk through the night by thousands of women in their bras! It proved to be an instant success, and eventually it became an annual event. To date she has raised over £83 million. It is a stunning success story and she has been cancer-free for many years, during which time she has married and had a beautiful little girl.

The financial state of our Centre had always been hazardous, and it took some years to gain real fundraising skills. The bulk of our original debt had been paid off by selling part of the Centre's original home in Downfield Road with planning consent for a number of small houses and, after Tim had died, selling the Old Rectory, the house that Christopher had bought for Mystica and him to retire to. The property boom meant that the Old Rectory, which had been modestly priced at purchase, had become enormously more valuable when it was sold. Christopher donated the house to the Centre just before sale so that it was free of capital gains tax. In spite of these windfalls, we were always struggling to balance the books. Now the wonderful Nina Barough was offering to help and we were able to increase the number of courses that we could offer clients.

I remember vividly the intense relief that Christopher and I felt when the bank finally returned the deeds of our personal house, which we had mortgaged in order to buy Grove House. We had been extraordinarily foolhardy to put our only home at jeopardy; if the Centre had failed it would have taken our home with it. Now, fortunately, all was well.

I remember being alone in the chapel at Grove House late one evening, after locking the place up and turning off the lights. I sat in meditation for a while and then spoke my intense thanks to God for this delivery. What a long, hard road it had been. If we had known how difficult it was going to be, would we have had the courage to do it? Then in my prayers I began to say, "And if you ever want us to move and buy another place, you are going to have to make it all a lot easier!" I seemed to hear the music of the old Scottish song "Oh, you'll take the high road, and I'll take the low road..." and the thought came to me: there is an easy way to do this and there is a hard way. We had just completed the hard way and should we ever need to embark on such foolishness again, we must find the easy way.

Some time later staff began to grumble that it was impossible to do all the things they wanted to do in Grove House because of lack of room. Would it be possible to build on another wing? Space was limited and although we did sketch out a plan, it didn't look the way to proceed. Trustees took up the question at board meetings. My heart sank. Did they know what they were suggesting? Every now and then one of them would come along with a great property that was coming onto the market. Would we go and visit it? I really didn't want to, but went along if only to say it was impossible. We passed over a number of properties and none of them came anywhere near what we were looking for.

Then one day a friend in the property business came along and asked a few of us to accompany him to see the old isolation hospital, Ham Green House at Pill, just outside Bristol. Dilapidated as it was, even I could see and feel that this was right for us. I stood on its steps and asked the question, "Is this where we are meant to be?" and I clearly and distinctly heard "Yes!" At last we were being shown our future home.

There were five acres of land that went down to the river. It was absolutely beautiful and full of potential. We inspected every nook and cranny and all came back with a resounding "Yes". There would be no difficulty, we were told, in pulling down all the NHS buildings and using the brown field site to build a purpose-built clinic. In addition, the old house would need to be upgraded and carefully restored. All we had to do was to acquire all the permissions and to find the seriously large amount of money that it would cost. Nina Barough was given a conducted tour and, while she was not in a position to promise, nevertheless she gave us encouragement to begin the process of purchase and planning.

Of course we used all our skills at fundraising, but we would never have had the courage to move forward if it hadn't been for Nina. I thought of the moment in the chapel, the high road and the low road: the easy way and the difficult way, and I was overwhelmed by a sense of gratitude for the help we were being offered. Our Patron, Prince Charles, was very involved in the design of the new buildings. We would go with the architect to Highgrove and lay out the plans on the table. It was impressive to see how informed and knowledgeable His Royal Highness was, and we made a number of changes to include his suggestions.

The whole scheme seemed to take a tremendously long time, but finally we moved into our new home in November 2006, and Prince Charles came to officially open it the following July. Like us he was thrilled with the twenty-six en-suite bedrooms, the many therapy rooms, meeting rooms, great dining room and lecture hall. The gardens were tenderly coaxed back to beauty and great windows allowed the light to stream in with wonderful vistas of garden and countryside at every turn. It was beautiful beyond our dreams and every part of it was shot through with transcendent glory. What an amazing place, but what should we call it? The idea grew that there was only one name that would do it justice: Penny Brohn Cancer Care.

The day we moved in I broke away from the celebrations to sit alone in the sanctuary. In the peace and stillness of the Centre I spoke to Penny, and sat there feeling her presence. Always when she and I had momentous, life-changing meetings in the past, beginning with her little room at Dr Issel's clinic in Germany and afterwards in many different places, she would break off from talking to point to a butterfly that was unaccountably flying above our heads, whatever time of year. It was our symbol of the heavenly presence of angels and helpers. Now, as I sat in gratitude in the sanctuary on this first day of our new life, I looked up to the rafters and beams and saw a beautiful butterfly circling round and round. It was the signal I was looking for and tears ran down my cheeks. Penny was here. Her world and ours were very close together, and at last we had come home. All was well.

• • • • • • •

Seventeen years had passed since Penny left us. I think constantly of how amazed and delighted she would be if she could wander around our beautiful new Centre with its enclosed courtyard garden, fountains sparkling in the sunlight and its elegant Georgian wing overlooking acres of landscaped parkland. Everything is here to ease the heart and delight the eye. Stress and tension drain away as our guests come through the door and take in the charm and beauty that awaits them. "You and I have got to change the world," Penny had said to me back in 1979, and the wonderful thing is that we have - the cancer world has indeed changed. There is a new understanding about the importance of quality of life and how it impacts survival. The 'Living Well' programme[27] was launched in November 2012 at the House of Commons in the presence of a large number of senior representatives from medicine and nursing. They were full of approval that we were taking our programme around the country, reaching thousands more people.

Chapter 16
The Golden Thread

Thirty years ago we were laughed at for wanting to take a body/mind/spirit approach, and now things are different. "With your thoughts you make the world", Buddha taught, and my heart misses a beat when I consider what we have done. Then it beats faster than ever when my mind considers what power we have, if we only know how to use it. Jesus spoke of moving mountains with our faith and belief. I have always assumed this was faith in Him and belief in His power. Supposing instead He was speaking of our power and our belief in our own ability to change the world. That would indeed be a message for this and future generations.

Religion has taught us that the power is beyond us, separate from us, yet so many people have had mystical experiences that suggest it is within; in an Oxford University study over 60% of people spoke of having a sense of the numinous, an 'otherness' that touched them with the glow of divinity[28]. It is this concept of interweaving divinity that made me call this book *The Golden Thread*. As I said at the beginning, the more we look for the grace and design in this world, the more we see it.

Clients tell me all the time of the synchronistic events that they become aware of after spending time at our Centre. I tell them that it happens all the time, only now they are becoming more aware. The more they notice, the more it will happen. I tell them that I believe in angels and that they exist to be our helpers.

"Ask for what you want," I say, "they need to be asked because they mustn't interfere unasked."

Is it true that angels exist? They have been part of inherited religious traditions for thousands of years, but who knows? If we find a concept or image helpful, then use the picture that comes to mind. If we don't, then use another image. It may well be that the power actually comes directly from us, but it takes an image to mobilise it. In science an experiment is valid if it can be repeated. If synchronicity works for you, then it is valid in the same way. In the Oxford study, when people wrote in detail of what they had experienced, the religious responders had figures from the faith they followed; non-religious responders had a sense of universal power confirming the oneness of all beings of nature and cosmic energy. We respond to things in our own way.

From the moment our embryonic cells start to beat, the heart engages with universal life and pulsing divinity. As the mind develops there grows a sense of connectedness and we want to know how we fit in to the scheme of things. At last we ask the essential questions: who am I and for what purpose was I born? This is the moment of awakening and the beginning of our great quest. Sooner or later a response begins to form. Love is the answer to both questions. We have come to give and receive love.

• • • • • • •

And now, as I draw towards the end of this book, I want to speak directly to you, dear reader, who have journeyed with me thus far.

You are conscious of the spiritual path that you are treading, or you would not have started and continued to read. Something has stirred in you that is leading you on, and it is to that essence of your being that I want to connect with now. All life, as I see it, is the journey of the soul. Every circumstance in our lives is grist to this mill: everything is a learning experience and educates the soul in one way or another. Nothing is wasted and no one is counting. It is entirely a personal matter how we educate our soul.

Returning to the other world, as I believe we do at the end of life, we will see how our life impacted on those around us. We may also make a list of the things that still need attention and determine to discover ways of working to improve in these areas. In that glorious place of light and love, it is easy to see that everything is connected; that all is one; that life goes on; that death is not the end and our essence and consciousness move back to what we experience as 'home'.

Is all this true? It is as true as anything else we have been told, because we have no way of measuring absolute and infinite truth. It is certainly as true as any religious teaching that may have come your way, and as good a guide for positive living. In the long run, all is metaphor and story to guide our thoughts and kindle our imaginations. It encapsulates one form of truth and relays it to us with a resonance that we can recognise.

People around us will have their personal metaphors and stories that work for them. We are all different and there is no one right and singular way. Once you remove dogma and judgement from the scenario, you see a wonderful flexibility that frees us to be ourselves. The yardstick by which we measure is love. In perplexity we ask, "What would Love do now?" and the way opens up. Jesus' final instruction to his friends was "Love one another as I have loved you." Words spoken as death is approaching have a particular significance and power, and words listened to by loved ones at such a time become beacons to guide the future. If we were taught this simple truth, "love one another as I have loved you" in infancy, what a difference it would make to the game of life. We would no longer ask: what is the point of trying when death ends all? We would understand that each life event has value, whether good or bad, because it presents an opportunity to practise courage, patience, endurance and self-control - all soul strengths that will not be lost.

Great spiritual teachers throughout the ages have taught that compassion - love in action - holds the universe together. Waking up to this, becoming aware, conscious and attentive, has led countless millions of devoted souls to move from the comfort of home to go out in selfless service to help the suffering. Our news broadcasts are full of terror and disaster, but countering that all over the world are the countless brave, good people who devote themselves wholeheartedly to answering the needs of the afflicted. They bridge the inner and the outer worlds without ego or judgement, answering the call of Love.

The sacred is in every breath of life. We see that as the wave cannot be separate from the ocean, so we cannot be separate from each other because all is one. And what of the age-old concept of God? God the creator, God the sustainer, God the judge? As we begin to accept that the quantum energetic field is everywhere, including in all sentient beings, then we might conceive that what has been known in the past as a particular god is actually the dynamic force that holds all things together, a force that is personal and universal at the same time. People who truly embody this source energy vibrate at a tremendously high level: the level of unconditional love. They are leading the world in spiritual awakening.

You, dear reader, are clearly on your way. You have persevered to the end of this book and I wish you joy as you travel on. Quantum science tells us that where particles are ever joined, they remain in touch and affected by each other. I who write this and you who read it are now joined. Together we move on to build a personal spiritual practice into our daily life, by meditating, by practising gratitude and compassion, by recognising source energy in nature, in the animal kingdom, in the food we eat and in the company of others on the journey.

Continue with or create any spiritual practice that resonates with you, explore it, build on it and see it now shot through with Divine energy that holds all things together. The heart needs to be engaged to put fire and warmth into the words. If you find yourself asking "Is it true?" and "Should I believe it?" the answer is that if it works for you and makes your heart beat faster and brings the tears to your eyes then it is true.

One Jewish writer put it this way: "I asked for God, and Jesus showed up!"[29] We need the personal and the particular. I was brought up Christian and married a Christian priest. It works for me, but so does the broader picture. I hold them both together in my heart, together with imagined angels and 'the whole company of heaven' of which my own dear Christopher is now one. It doesn't have to make sense, it just has to work for me.

Do not expect everyone to understand. People live in their own mythical world and yet they want a general theory that will cover everything. In fact we dwell in multiple parallel universes, each encapsulated within our own belief bubble. There is no valid language that can unite them all. Our consciousness is intimate, unique and continuous and body and mind are interacting moment by moment in an ongoing and mysterious dance. Einstein's colleague Max Planck said "When you change the way you look at things, the things you are looking at change."[30]

May this change renew, restore and revitalise you and may every blessing be yours.

> They said, "You have a blue guitar.
> You do not play things as they are."
> The man replied, "Things as they are
> Are changed upon a blue guitar."

Wallace Stevens[31]

A last word from Pat. This piece was written as a possible preface to the book and sent to her publisher in the final month of her life.

On the last day of June 2012, as I was travelling to France for a lovely holiday with my daughter and grand-daughter, I missed my footing on a speed bump and landed on my hip. So instead of France, it was blue-lighting by ambulance to hospital for the first time in my 83 years! The message from the universe was clear: I was grounded for a purpose, and that was to get on with the book. It was a shock, of course, but I was not surprised. The hip mended and life went on, but I could tell that something had changed. Eventually weight loss took me to my doctor and the medical process was set in motion which finally revealed that I had an inoperable pancreatic tumour and just a few weeks to live.

People who know me well and understand my deepest thoughts have known of my longing to go home to Christopher, my husband of fifty four years. He died in 2007 and I have enjoyed a very good life in his absence but always ached to be with him. Now I have been given my passport to take my leave and return to a world that is familiar and longed for, and where he is waiting with open arms. So as I write this in the August of 2013, I am in the waiting room of the outer courts of heaven, and I am absolutely content. My family are all around me, my closest friends are here and I have all I need to stay in my own beautiful home, enjoying the summer roses, the banks of lavender and the glades of trees in full, magnificent bloom.

My heart reaches out to you who have read this book. I hope it has answered some of your questions, and that you will understand that the vital thing to know is that the soul is eternal, and life goes on. Energy is never lost: it always reforms. Soul energy is the essence and source of our being. Nothing of value in me is being lost now. It will be there around you, in the wind, in the stars and in everything you love and cherish, until in the fullness of time we are reunited once again.

Pat Pilkington
August 2013

Reflections on the final weeks of Pat's life, written by her daughter, Felicity Biggart

In this book my mother has recorded many strands of wisdom and teaching that weave together to make up the spiritual golden thread that ran through both her life and my father's. It was an extraordinary journey from the life of a vicar's wife to the founding of a holistic cancer help centre, extending help, love and care to so many people. Her own final months on this earth are also a remarkable part of this journey, bearing so many parallels to the stories and teaching within *The Golden Thread* and I would like to share my experience of this final chapter of my mother's life.

My mother's physical decline began in the last days of June 2012, in her eighty-third year. My daughter, my mother and I had set out in the early morning to begin a two-week stay at our holiday home in the mountains of Provence.

As we waited at the Channel Tunnel terminal, she fell on a raised walkway, breaking her hip. Rather than spending a pleasant evening at the hotel we had booked near Beaune, we found ourselves in a state of shock at Ashford Hospital.

With her typical stoic determination she was up and about and walking again in a very short period of time. As ever, she searched for meaning in life events and found the positive answer. Her first action was to ensure she was present again at Penny Brohn, to provide her inspirational talks. Her second was to begin writing this book.

A little more than a year after the fall I was once again planning to leave for two weeks in France. Before going I visited my mother to say a temporary goodbye. I remember the garden filled with sunshine, birdsong and roses; the stillness and the warm light of a perfect summer's day. I remember my mother, backlit by this glory, as we sat together on her patio.

We knew that my mother, who had always been so strong, had been rendered fragile by something affecting her digestion. She had lost a lot of weight, and her arms, exposed for the first time in short sleeves, were alarmingly thin. However, as far as we knew, all the tests and explorations had not found anything wrong. She reassured me all was well and turned the conversation to other matters. With a lovely smile and a warm hug she waved me away.

With my two children, Matthew and Rachael, I drove across France. Early on our first morning at our holiday home, we went down to the lake to swim and shake off the long journey. On our return, my mother telephoned. "My darling girl, I have pancreatic cancer and I am going to die."

My children sat with their arms around me and we cried. And I wondered what on earth had possessed my mother, just three days earlier, to let me leave for France. With cheeks still wet I sat down at the computer and booked a flight home.

After a colonoscopy had found nothing awry, my mother's consultant had turned his attention to the upper tract of her digestive system. He had arranged a scan. She had received the results before our last meeting in the garden. Why she had withheld this news, I can only speculate. On a conscious level she said that she had wanted us all to have our holiday, but perhaps she needed time for her own reflection, uninterrupted by our pain and distress.

Now I have come to know this book so well I can suggest another interpretation of her silence. She was preparing herself for a conscious leave taking from this world. On almost every page of this book there is a message that we have choice, that you can choose your path even in the final stages of illness, including choosing when it is right to go. The story of Father Andrew in chapter 13, which had so comforted both my parents, is a direct parallel to my mother's departure. Both she and Father Andrew faced the inevitability of their death without fear and made choices about how they would die.

And so I arrived home to be with my mother, with no intent to leave again for as long as she needed me. We thought we had a few months, but in fact the final step in the path took only ten days. I watched as she stepped into that active space of preparing for her own transition from this world into the next, something she had been preparing for over all the years of her deep study and reflection.

As we sat together once again in the beauty of her lovely home, she held my hand and said that her last gift to us all was to teach us how to die well. For so many years the message she had offered at Penny Brohn was how to live well with cancer; yet also, as she talked with the clients, opening up the possibilities of the healing space of the spirit, she shared with them the beauty and grace that might be found on leaving this world, and the possibility of our life's endeavour continuing into the next. I have found this last gift to us to be a joyous one, taking away many of my fears of death and dying. Indeed, she shared these very words with my brother John, in July, passing on Tim's teaching for the final time:

This is what Tim told us: there comes a point in dying when you are in your disintegrating body and there are actually now two of you. The one that steps out feels completely vigorous and has no interest in the one that is lying on the bed. All negativity is attached to the physical body.

What those sitting around the bed see as a last breathing out, in the new spiritual body, is a first gulp of fresh air, and the embrace of loved and long lost friends.

So the person leaving doesn't experience being dead. But those sitting around do. Sometimes those sitting experience the first part of the journey, rising with the person and seeing the welcoming committee and seeing the person who has been so diminished vigorous and full of life and greeting long lost friends.

Then they return and after a period of quiet one will say to the other: I've just had the strangest experience, the other person says I have too, and they share the experience. And the hospice carer, standing in the background, says that this happens all the time.

My mother, showing a determination that was stoic, magical, inspiring and terrifying, began to jump out of her body in such huge leaps that each day we saw the change. Not the change in her spirit, but the change in her body. And as the strength in her physical body declined there was a corresponding growth in her spiritual presence.

When I arrived for this last stage, she could still walk to the door and appreciate the beauty of her garden. In the morning, after her shower, she would sit in her chair in her sun-filled kitchen. Her house brought her such joy, she had created and designed it with my father. My memories of this time are shot through with an exquisite light shining upon us all. There was something magical in the air, as if the universe were blessing us with the best it could offer.

Elaine. No story of my mother's life and death would be complete without a mention of the wonderful Elaine, who had been my father's carer and companion and then my mother's housekeeper. She was a trained auxiliary nurse and was on leave from her usual job, due to an injury. She could not do the heavy lifting demanded by her own job – but she had the skill to guide us as we learned how to hold and care for my mother. More than this she bought us the gift of her singing voice: pure, beautiful and uplifting.

And so, on her final day, I watched my mother depart, in the middle of all this glory and sunshine, with the garden in full bloom. She was surrounded by love. Absolutely surrounded by it, because she had given so generously throughout her life.

This was reflected so beautifully in His Royal Highness Prince Charles's thoughtful words following her death. His obituary (which we reproduce here in full) exactly captures the essence of all Penny and my mother created, inspired by the depth of this faith and belief in the healing power of love. As a family we were delighted to have such a wonderful acknowledgement of my mother's work from someone she regarded as a friend, as well as the highly valued patron of the charity she gave her life to.

It was my great good fortune to have known Pat Pilkington for the best part of thirty years, and to have seen at first hand how her boundless energy, spirit and positive outlook helped to transform the quality of so many lives through her work with Penny Brohn Cancer Care formerly known as the Bristol Cancer Help Centre.

I met Pat on several occasions, together with her husband, Christopher, who was a huge supporter of all that she did and I remember being incredibly impressed by their passion and commitment when I opened the charity's new premises at Clifton, in 1983. There was a real sense of pioneering work that they both espoused and I greatly admired what she achieved with a genuinely integrated approach to the care of cancer sufferers.

Pat, and Penny Brohn herself, always emphasised the importance of treating the whole person - something we often talked about.

Today, managing the impact of a cancer diagnosis, offering advice and help with vital elements such as nutrition and providing emotional and spiritual support, are all part of the complementary provision at Penny Brohn Cancer Care, which I have seen for myself, and for which we owe a huge debt of gratitude to Pat.

· · · · · · ·

I do not know what awaits us after death or in the next world, but I do know that my mother chose to go in her own time and way. Everything happened as she had asked. My two wonderful brothers, Mark and John; her closest companions and friends – we were each able to give all that she wanted us to give. She was filled with an absolute belief of an onward journey and a glorious homecoming, a reunion with everyone she loved. In every moment and nuance of that final day, there was a quiet perfection.

Whilst I was still in France, Mum had sent me an email saying, "Yours is the hand I want to hold as I go." No easy task given that she also said that she did not want any deathbed vigils. She wanted peace to pray and meditate and prepare herself.

I need not have worried. Somehow we all knew when the exact moment had arrived. As I sat with her I reached for her hand. I felt hers close within mine, so I know she was aware of my presence. In the kitchen across the hall Elaine began to sing in her beautiful pure voice. As the first song ended, I felt again the slight tensing in Mum's hand. Then seamlessly Elaine moved from one uplifting song to the next, the most beautiful serenade.

And so, on the gentle summer's evening of 19th August 2013, my mother relaxed and let go of this life, and with arms wide open stepped from this world to the next and is now, I am sure, with her beloved Christopher.

Felicity Biggart, January 2015

Remembering Pat, by Michael Connors, Director of Services, Penny Brohn Cancer Care

As Director of Services at Penny Brohn I am delighted that Pat found the time and strength needed to complete this book in the final year of her life. As I read it again I am struck by the memory of my last time with Pat at our national Centre near Bristol in the summer of 2013.

On our 'Approach' residential course we gather our clients together for an evening talk. These occasions offer the clients an opportunity to reflect, contemplate and enquire on some of the bigger questions that a diagnosis of cancer asks of them and their loved ones. Pat used to lead these conversations and clients found them deeply moving.

Pat had told me that she was dying and that this would be her last talk so I attended. It was a warm July evening and I met Pat at reception and we both went into the room together. We waited for the group to arrive and chatted and laughed together. I noted that she was in very good spirits even though her body was frail and that, still, her eyes shone with such intensity and passion.

Sitting beside her I was struck by all Pat represented. She was from a generation that had broken the ground in spirituality and I realised she was now handing on the baton to a new era of care at the Centre. She was quite direct in telling me that this was her intention: she wanted us to carry forward the work that she and many others had helped to create.

It was not Pat's way to take the easy path. She could have spent her life fully occupied in being, as she put it, 'a Church of England minister's wife'. However, both Christopher and Pat wanted to explore so much more within their ministry. While not personally losing their deep Christian faith they offered an enquiry into a new space of all faiths and none, and into personal spirituality and holistic thinking, that for its time was very radical. Pat's core tenet was that the restoration of the spirit was an essential part of holistic healing.

When the group arrived we sat for a moment in silence and mindfulness and then Pat began the conversation with stories of her life and the creation of the Centre.

These evening sessions offered Pat an opportunity to share her thoughts, understandings, experiences and passion for spirituality. She would offer her words voluntarily from her deep commitment to this enquiry and with a fascination with the deepest human questions. She loved that science was exploring the edge of mystery and she was always full of the latest research from new books and papers that were showing how we as humans are much more than just a mechanistic process, how there was some grand design and a greater intelligence at work.

What happens in death? Where have we come from? Who am I now after this journey? What really matters? How can I be an active part in my healing and recovery? How can I feel whole again?

These sorts of questions are brought into sharp relief by the journey that cancer patients must endure. Pat knew, of course, that there are no absolutes in answering these questions, however, this never stopped her highlighting the importance of this opportunity to enquire into them.

I remember at the end being moved deeply by the conversation, the strength of Pat's conviction, the openness of the clients and the clear sense that the discussions were, and remain, at the heart of the Penny Brohn Whole Person Approach.

In her talk that night, Pat offered an open acceptance for all approaches to spirituality and explored the concept of the Golden Thread: that a mysterious core sits at the heart of all religions and indeed within the heart of us all. She offered the symbology of poetry, prayer and story to highlight some of the possible enquiries into this mystery and listened to the clients as they shared their experiences, beliefs, fears, wisdoms and personal understandings. She did this with compassion and empathic warmth, which radiated acceptance and interest in what was being said.

At the end Pat offered a prayer and her familiar Buddhist blessing: "May you be happy" and we sat in a profound silence again.

By the end of the enquiry many of the clients said that they now felt that some deep hope had been re-enlivened. Not a false hope about cure, or that everything is OK, but a hope that there is a greater purpose, a deeper meaning, a reprioritising and another way forward in their lives. This of course resonates with all of the services at Penny Brohn, which are offered to help and support people to find what they need to progress in their ability to live well with the impact of cancer.

I walked with Pat to the door at the end and we said our goodbyes and she offered a hug as she always did. She stood for the last time in her beloved beautiful centre, which now offers support to thousands of people, and has services that blossomed here in Bristol, reaching across the UK.

She stood at the entrance absorbing the ambience that she always described as feeling like a loving embrace for all who arrive. This magnificent place that began as a dream around a table in Bristol where a charity was formed that has journeyed, like us all, through times of ease and times of crisis. This place that was her greatest gift and at times her greatest burden. She stood smiling, eyes still filled with life and hope, even in the full knowledge of her coming death.

As I think about this now I think of her saying:

"My dear Michael, you know faith really can move mountains!"

I wrote a poem soon after that last evening together. She had planted three trees in memory of Christopher; his favourite paper birches. As a Canon of the Church of England he was very important in the development of Penny Brohn Cancer Care's spiritual openness and acceptance of all faiths and none.

In her talks and through her connections with clients Pat offered so much hope, compassion and wise words. This helped our clients find the meaning, the inspiration and resources to find their way through sometimes very difficult terrain. This poem highlights that one of her great offerings was the knowledge that there is always hope.

Remembering the dawn

There is always the night,
when the remembering of your sunny day has past
and now the lighted windows spill across the lawn,

This garden, full and rich, embraces a welcome
for the ones who come to find a way through the dark.

At the entrance, three trees, young and strong, birch, white paper peeled,
planted for a beloved one.
A moment's breeze moves them,
and they bow to those hearts that opened, hands that built, minds
that knew and souls that led to here.

At times like this the heart can feel a silent dread,
for there is not even a moon to light the way,
the dark only a reminder of the fear,
stirring the cry of a wounded life, a lost opportunity;
the gift that lies waiting to be opened.

But in this time, I will always see through the lighted window, a
room, 10 souls gathered, her body frail but eyes filled with the fire

of truth and love.
Voice lifted by the passion of heart and conviction of soul.
Reminding us, reminding us of who we really are and how we still have time,
to find what we know we must find and what we think we have lost.

Soothing the hearts that fear

Her words point through this darkest hour,
trusting something more than this,
reminding us to know

"The dawn will always come, the dawn will always come."

As her hand clasps her beloved's hand, at the white birch trees,
in the east a soft light is opening.

Learning to Live Well

Penny Brohn Cancer Care has led the way in a whole person approach to cancer for over thirty years. From its earliest days as the Bristol Cancer Help Centre, it has helped thousands of people take back control of their health and wellbeing and support their own healing process.

Penny Brohn's Whole Person Approach recognises that there is more to health than what happens in our physical bodies. It recognises that to be resilient and to function as well as we can in any situation, we also need to pay attention to our mental, emotional and spiritual health because they are all closely connected.

The Whole Person Approach supports health in each of these different areas to give the best chance of living as well as possible for as long as possible. It has been designed to help people at each stage of their cancer experience and works alongside medical and other cancer treatments.

Penny Brohn provide a range of services, including residential and day courses, which are free of charge to adults with a cancer diagnosis and their supporters. They offer self help techniques and complementary therapies as well as lifestyle measures such as healthy eating, physical activity and ways of managing stress and difficult emotions.

The charity relies on funding and donations to enable it to continue to reach more and more people affected by cancer. To find out how to support their life changing work contact fundraising@pennybrohn.org.

Penny Brohn Cancer Care
Chapel Pill Lane, Pill, Bristol, BS20 0HH
Telephone: 01275 370 100 | Email: info@pennybrohn.org
www.pennybrohncancercare.org
Registered Charity no. 284881

References

1   Stephen Hawking, *A Brief History of Time*, Bantam, 2000

2   Frank Morison, *Who moved the Stone?* Authentic Media, 2006

3   We do not know which edition Pat used, but you might try Lynn Bauman, *The Gospel of Thomas: The Wisdom of the Twin*, White Cloud Press, 2012

4   Wayne Dyer, *The Power of Intention: Learning to Co-create the World in Your Way*, Hay House , 2004

5   From the *Dhammapada*. We do not know which translation Pat used. You might try Gil Fronsdal, *Dhammapada*, Shambhala 2006

6   Caroline Myss, *Entering the Castle: An Inner Path to God and Your Soul*, Simon and Schuster Ltd, 2007

7   The Bible: John 8:32

8   ibid

9   The Bible: John 4:34

10   Caroline Myss, *Invisible Acts of Power*, Scribner, 2006

11   Guy Brown, *The Energy of Life*, Flamingo, 2000

12   John Robinson, *Honest to God, 50th Anniversary Edition*, SCM Press, 2013

13   Elizabeth Kubler-Ross, *On Life After Death*, Celestial Arts, 1991/2008

14   Jonathan Dimbleby, *The Prince of Wales*, Harper Collins, 1996

15   Joseph Chiltern Pearce, *The Biology of Transcendence*, Park Street Press, 2004

16   Susan Jeffers, *Feel the Fear and Do It Anyway*, Vermillion, 2007

17   Pat Rodegast, *Emmanuel's Book*, Bantam Doubleday, 1987

18   Raymond A Moody, *Glimpses of Eternity*, Rider, 2011

19   Rodegast, ibid

20   Rupert Sheldrake, *Dogs That Know When Their Owners Are Coming Home*, Arrow, 2000

21   Timothy Freke, *The Mystery Experience*, Watkins, 2012

22   From *The History of Penny Brohn Cancer Care*, a booklet published by Penny Brohn Cancer Care and written by Mark Seymour.

23   Penny Brohn, *Gentle Giants*, Ebury Press, 1987

24   Philip Larkin, *The North Ship*, Faber & Faber, 1987

25   Danah Zohar, *Spiritual Intelligence*, Bloomsbury, 2001

26   Caroline Myss, *Sacred Contracts: Awakening Your Divine Potential*, Bantam, 2002

27   For further information on the 'Living Well' programme, see www.pennybrohncancercare.org/living-well

28   David Hay, *Religious Experience Today: Studying the Facts*, Mowbray, 1990. David Hay was Director of the Religious Experience Research Unit at the University of Oxford and carried out many studies testing human spiritual awareness.

29   I'm afraid we have no idea who Pat was referring to here, despite searching the internet and asking her friends. We wanted to leave in the quote, to be true to Pat's words.

30   Quote widely attributed to Max Planck, source unknown.

31   Wallace Stevens, *Collected Poems*, Faber & Faber, 2006

Bibliography

These books were all found in Pat's library, and are listed here as a source of reference for those who might like to explore further some of the ideas in this book.

Eban Alexander, *Proof of Heaven: A Neurosurgeon's Journey into the Afterlife*, Piatkus, 2012
Karen Armstrong, *The Case for God*, Vintage, 2010
Karen Armstrong, *Twelve Steps to a Compassionate Life*, Bodley Head, 2011
Coleman Barks, *Rumi: Bridge to the Soul: Journeys into the Music and Silence of the Heart*, HarperOne, 2007
Richard Bartlett, *Matrix Energetics: The Science and Art of Transformation*, Beyond Words Publishing, 2009
Richard Bartlett, *The Physics of Miracles: Tapping into the Field of Consciousness Potential*, Beyond Words Publishing, 2010
William Bloom, *The Power of Modern Spirituality*, Piatkus, 2011
William Bloom, *The Endorphin Effect: A Breakthrough Strategy for Holistic Health and Spiritual Wellbeing*, Piatkus, 2011
Gregg Braden, *The Divine Matrix: Bridging Time, Space, Miracles and Belief*, Hay House UK, 2008
Gregg Braden, *Secrets of the Lost Mode of Prayer*, Hay House UK, 2006
Gregg Braden, *The Spontaneous Healing of Belief*, Hay House, 2008
Isobel Briggs Myers, *Gifts Differing: Understanding Personality Types*, Davies-Black Publishing, 1995
Penny Brohn, *Gentle Giants: A Powerful Story of One Woman's Unconventional Struggle against Breast Cancer*, Ebury Press, 1987
Rhonda Byrne, *The Secret*, Simon and Schuster Ltd, 2006
Richard Carlson, *Handbook for The Soul: A Collection of Writings on Spirituality*, Piatkus, 1996
Dolores Cannon, *Jesus and the Essenes*, Ozark Mountain Publishing, 2000
Joseph Chiltern Pearce, *The Biology of Transcendence: A Blueprint of the Human Spirit*, Park Street Press, USA, 2004
Joseph Chiltern Pearce, *Heart-Mind Matrix: How the Heart Can Teach the Mind New Ways to Think*, Park Street Press reprint, 2012

Joseph Chiltern Pearce, *Death of Religion and the Rebirth of Spirit*, Park Street Press , 2007

Deepak Chopra, *Quantum Healing: Exploring the Frontiers of Mind, Body and Spirit*, Bantam, 1989

Deepak Chopra, *Perfect Health*, Bantam, 2001

Deepak Chopra, *The Deeper Wound: Preserving Your Soul in the Face of Fear and Tragedy*, Rider, 2012

Deepak Chopra, *The Third Jesus: How to Find Truth and Love in Today's World*, Rider, 2009

Deepak Chopra, *Life After Death: The Book of Answers*, Rider, 2008

Deepak Chopra, *The Book of Secrets: Who am I? Where did I come from? Why am I here?* Rider, 2004

Deepak Chopra, *How to Know God: The Soul's Journey into the Mystery of Mysteries*, Rider, 2001

Deepak Chopra, *Synchrodestiny: Harnessing the Infinite Power of Coincidence*, Rider, 2005

Deepak Chopra, *Reinventing the Body, Resurrecting the Soul*, Rider, 2011

Deepak Chopra, *Molecules of Emotion: Why you Feel the Way You Do* (with Candice Pert), Pocket Books, 1999

Dawson Church, *The Genie in Your Genes*, Energy Psychology Press, 2009

Rosy Daniel, *The Cancer Prevention Book: A Complete Mind/Body Approach* (with Rachael Ellis), Hunter House Publishing, 2002

Rosy Daniel, *The Cancer Directory: A Mine of Information on the Latest Orthodox and Complementary Treatments*, Harper Thorsons, 2005

Rosy Daniel, *Living with Cancer,* Robinson, 2000

Larry Dossey, *Reinventing Medicine: Beyond Mind-Body into a New Era of Healing*, HarperOne, 2000

Larry Dossey, *Healing Beyond the Body: Medicine and the Infinite Reach of the Mind*, Piatkus, 2009

Larry Dossey, *Be Careful What You Pray For; You Just Might Get It*, HarperSanFrancisco, 1998

Larry Dossey, *Recovering the Soul: A Scientific and Spiritual Search*, Bantam Doubleday, 1997

Larry Dossey, *Prayer is Good Medicine: How to Reap the Benefits of Prayer,* HarperSanFrancisco, 1997

Larry Dossey, *One Mind: We are Part of a Greater Consciousness. Does it matter?.* Hay House, 2013

Larry Dossey, *Space. Time and Medicine*, Shambhala, 1982

Larry Dossey, *Beyond Illness: Discovering the Experience of Health*, Shambala, 1991

Larry Dossey, *Healing Words*, HarperOne, 1995

Larry Dossey, *Meaning and Medicine: Lessons from a Doctor's Tales of Breakthrough and Healing*, Bantam Doubleday, 1997

Wayne Dyer, *The Power of Intention: Learning to Co-create the World in Your Way*, Hay House , 2004

Wayne Dyer, *There is a Spiritual Solution to Every Problem*, Hay House UK, 2002

Wayne Dyer, *A New Way of Thinking: A New Way of Being*, Hay House UK, 2010

Gill Edwards, *Life is a Gift: A Practical Guide to Making Your Dreams Come True*, Piatkus, 2007

Gill Edwards, *Stepping into the Magic: A New Approach to Everyday Life*, Piatkus, 2010

Gill Edwards, *Wild Love*, Piatkus, 2009

Gill Edwards, *Conscious Medicine: Creating Health and Wellbeing in a Conscious Universe*, Piatkus, 2010

Charles Foster, *Wired for God: The Biology of Spiritual Experience*, Hodder and Stoughton, 2011

Matthew Fox, *The Coming of the Cosmic Christ*, Harper One, 1990

Matthew Fox, *Original Blessing: Primer in Creation Spirituality*, Bear and Company, 1987

Matthew Fox, *Western Spirituality*, Bear and Company, 1987

Matthew Fox, *Creation Spirituality*, Harper SanFrancisco, 1991

Matthew Fox, *The Hidden Spirituality of Men*, New World Library, 2009

Victor Frankl, *Man's Search for Meaning*, Rider, 2004

Barbara Fredrickson, *Positivity: Groundbreaking Research to Release Your Inner Optimist and Thrive*, One World Publications, 2011

Timothy Freke, *The Laughing Jesus* (with Peter Gandy), O Books, 2006

Timothy Freke, *Jesus and the Lost Goddess: The Secret Teachings of the Original Christians*, Harmony, 2008

Timothy Freke, *How Long Is Now? How to be Spiritually Awake in the Real World*, Hay House UK, 2009

Timothy Freke, *The Mystery Experience: A Revolutionary Approach to Spiritual Awakening*, Watkins, 2012

Robert Fritz, *The Path of Least Resistance: Learning to Become the Creative Force in Your Own Life*, DMA, 1984

Robert Fritz, *Creating*, Fawcett Books, 1991

Jane E Gillham, *The Science of Optimism and Hope: Research Essays*, Templeton Foundation, 2000

David Hamilton, *How Your Mind Can Heal Your Body*, Hay House UK, 2008

Stephen Hoeller, *Jung and the Lost Gospels*, Quest Books, USA, 1989

James Hillman, *The Soul's Code: In Search of Character and Calling*, Warner Books, 1996

James Hillman, *Re-visioning Psychology*, First Harper, 1977/1992

James Hillman, *A Blue Fire: Selected Writings*, Harper Perennial, 1991

Susan Jeffers, *Feel the Fear and Do It Anyway*, Vermillion, 2007

Elisabeth Kubler-Ross, *On Life After Death*, Celestial Arts, 1991/2008

Robert Lanza, *Biocentrism: How Life Creates the Universe, Not the Other Way Around*, Ben Bella, 2010

Lawrence LeShan, *You Can Fight for Your Life*, M Evans & Co, 1980

Lawrence LeShan, *The Mechanic and the Gardener*, Henry Holt, 1982

Lawrence LeShan, *Cancer as a Turning Point: Handbook for People with Cancer,* Penguin Books Ltd, 1989

Lawrence LeShan, *Landscapes of the Mind: The Faces of Reality*, Eirini Press, 2012

Bruce Lipton, *The Biology of Belief,* Hay House, 2005

Bruce Lipton, *The Honeymoon Effect: the Science of Creating Heaven on Earth*, Hay House UK, 2013

David Lorimer, *A New Renaissance: Transforming Science, Spirit and Society*, Floris Books, 2010

Diarmaid MacCulloch, *Christianity: The First Three Thousand Years*, Penguin Books, 2011

Iain Mcgilchrist, *The Master and His Emissary: The Divided Brain and the Making of the Western World,* Yale University Press, 2009

Lynne McTaggart, T*he Field: The Quest for the Secret Force of the Universe,* Element, 2003

Lynne McTaggart, *The Bond: Connecting Through the Space Between Us*, Hay House, 2011

Joanna Macy, *Active Hope: How to Face the Mess We're In Without Going Crazy* (with Chris Johnstone), New World Library, 2012

Barbara Marx Hubbard, *Emergence: The Shift from Ego to Essence*, Hampton Roads, 2001/2012

Barbara Marx Hubbard, *Conscious Evolution: Awakening the Power of Our Social Potential*, New World Library, 1998

Raymond A Moody, *Glimpses of Eternity: Shared Death Experiences*, Rider, 2011

Thomas Moore, *Care of the Soul: A Guide for Cultivating Depth and Sacredness in Everyday Life,* Harper Collins/Piatkus, 1992/2012

Thomas Moore, *Writing in the Sand: Jesus, Spirituality, and the Soul of the Gospels*, Hay House, 2009

Thomas Moore, *Care of the Soul in Medicine: Guidance for Patients and Those Who Care for Them*, Hay House UK, 2012

Thomas Moore, *Dark Nights of the Soul: A Guide to Finding your Way through Life's Ordeals*, Gotham Books, 2005

Thomas Moore, *The Soul's Religion*, Bantam, 2003

Anita Moorjani, *Dying to Be Me: My Journey from Cancer to Near Death to True Healing*, Hay House, 2012/2014

Caroline Myss, *Anatomy of the Spirit: The Seven Stages of Power and Healing,* Bantam, 1997

Caroline Myss, *Why People Don't Heal and How They Can*, Bantam, 1998

Caroline Myss, *Sacred Contracts: Awakening Your Divine Potential*, Bantam, 2002

Caroline Myss, *Defy Gravity: Healing Beyond the Bounds of Reason*, Bantam, 2009

Caroline Myss, *The Creation of Health: Merging Traditional Medicine with*

Intuitive Diagnosis (with Norman Shealy), Bantam, 1992

Caroline Myss, *Entering the Castle: An Inner Path to God and Your Soul*, Simon and Schuster Ltd, 2007

Michael Neill, *The Inside-Out Revolution*, Hay House, 2013

Michael Newton, *Journey of Souls: Case Studies of Life Between Lives*, Llewellyn Publications, 1994

Michael Newton, *Memories of the After Life: Stories of Personal Transformation*, Llewellyn Publications, 2009

Arnold M Patent, *You Can Have it All: Universal Principles in Action*, Beyond Words Publishing, 2001/2007

M S Richardson, *Energenics: The Life Force That Fills the Cosmos and Powers Creation*, Athena Press, 2012

Pat Rodegast, *Emmanuel's Book: A Manual for Living Comfortably*, Bantam Doubleday, 1987

Pat Rodegast, *A Choice for Love: Emmanuel's Book II*, Bantam Doubleday, 1989

Pat Rodegast, *Emmanuel's Book III: What Is An Angel Doing Here?*, Bantam Doubleday, 1994

Gary Schwartz, *The Afterlife Experiments: Breakthrough Scientific Evidence of Life After Death*, Simon and Schuster, 2002/2003

Gary Schwartz, *Sacred Promise: How Science is Discovering Spirit's Collaboration with us in our Daily Lives*, Beyond Words Publishing, 2011

Martin Seligman, *Learned Optimism: How to Change Your Mind and Your Life*, Vintage Books, USA, 2006

Martin Seligman, *Flourish: A New Understanding of Happiness and Wellbeing*, Nicholas Brealey, 2011

Martin Seligman, *What You Can Change and What You Can't*, Nicholas Brealey, 2007

Sky Shayne Innes, *Love's Alchemy: Extraordinary Awareness for Extraordinary Living*, Heartfelt Publishing, 2009

Norman Shealy, *Soul Medicine: Awakening your Blueprint for Abundant Health and Energy*, Elite Books, 2008

Rupert Sheldrake, *The Science Delusion*, Coronet, 2012

Rupert Sheldrake, *Dogs That Know When Their Owners Are Coming Home*, Arrow, 2000

Rupert Sheldrake, *The Presence of the Past: Morphic Resonance*, Icon Books Ltd, 2011

Graham Stanton, *Gospel Truth: The Quest for an Eye Witness to Christ*, Fount, 1997

Edmon, Szekely, *The Gospel of the Essenes*, C W Daniel Co Ltd, 1976

Steve Taylor, *Waking from Sleep: Why Awakening Experiences Occur and How to Make them Permanent*, Hay House UK, 2010

Eckhart Tolle, *The Power of Now: A Guide to Spiritual Enlightenment*, Hodder Paperbacks, 2001

Eckhart Tolle, *Stillness Speaks: Whispers of Now*, Hodder Mobius, 2003

Eckhart Tolle, *A New Earth: Create a Better Life*, Penguin, 2009

Frances Vaughan, *Shadows of the Sacred: Seeing Through Spiritual Illusions*, Backinprint.com, 2005

Frances Vaughan, *Awakening Intuition*, Anchor Books, 1988

Marianne Williamson, *A Return to Love: Reflections on 'A Course of Miracles'*, Thorsons, 1996

Marianne Williamson, *The Gift of Chang: Spiritual Guidance for a Radically New Life*, Element, 2011

Lisa Williams, *The Survival of the Soul*, Hay House UK, 2011

Mark Williams, *Mindfulness: A Practical Guide to Finding Peace in a Frantic World*, Piatkus, 2011

Danah Zohar, *Spiritual Intelligence: The Ultimate Intelligence*, Bloomsbury Publishing, 2001

Danah Zohar, *The Quantum Self: Quantum Psychology and Quantum Morality*, Flamingo, 1991

Gary Zukov, *The Seat of the Soul: An Inspiring Vision*, Rider, 1991

Gary Zukov, *Heart of the Soul*, Simon and Schuster, 2002

Gary Zukov, *Spiritual Partnership: The Journey to Authentic Power*, Rider, 2010

Gary Zukov, *The Dancing Wu Li Masters: An Overview of the New Physics*, Rider, 1991

Gary Zukov, *The Mind of the Soul*, Simon and Schuster Ltd, 2004

Acknowledgements

First I need to acknowledge the gift my mother gave me in asking me to ensure this wonderful book was published. To say she dedicated her life to helping others would be an understatement. She had an endless capacity to love that meant she could live her life no other way.

In writing these acknowledgements on her behalf I have yet again wrapped myself up in the memory of this love and hope that I do justice to her voice, and to her desire to thank the following people.

First and foremost I would like to thank my wonderful brothers, Mark and John, for their generosity in letting me take this book forward with their wholehearted support and the freedom to fulfil this last task for our mother. The loving generosity inherent within them reflects the warmth and love that filled our family home. The depth of their care was steadfast to the end of Mum's life and allowed her the gift of leaving this world joyously and without regret at the sorrow of those left behind.

In any acknowledgment of contribution to this book my mother would have placed Ashley and Michael Akin-Smith at the centre. What can I say of a friendship so deep and a love so abiding and a home as warm and welcoming as my mother's own? Mum spent many hours with Ashley and her glorious husband Michael, finding refuge and peace in their lovely home following the death of my father. She was ever the provider, but she would allow Michael and Ashley to enfold her with their care and feed her.

Pat and Ashley travelled a path together of shared joy in spiritual inquiry and learning. Books read in delight and inspiration, shared and challenged views, a friendship unaltered by the separation of death. This book could not have been published without Ashley's knowledge and understanding of my mother's spiritual philosophy and thought. It is a friendship that has held and sustained me through the process of editing and bringing this book to publication.

There are so many reasons for me to thank all the wonderful team at Penny Brohn Cancer Care, but in particular I would like to thank Laura Kerby, Michael Connors and Kathie Burton. They have given hours of time both reading the book and giving feedback and support. Michael has also offered us his own words for inclusion in the book, not to mention the gift of his creativity with his beautifully crafted poem inspired by my mother's living memorial for my father – the planting of three silver birch trees in the grounds of Penny Brohn.

I would also like to thank Kathie for the kind introduction to her friend and professional editor, Jackie King. Jackie holds the distinction of both having never met my mother, but knowing the beat of her heart and the inner eye of her spiritual journey. She has been a gift of kindness and professional excellence from the heavens, so in tune with my mother's belief that 'when you ask with clarity for what you need you will find it.' We did not know how to ask for Jackie, so I can only assume mum was part of the interviewing process in the next realm and in league with Kathie, sent us the perfect candidate. I only wish I had another book for her to edit.

During the last two years of her life my mother was determined that her spiritual work with clients would go on and that she could successfully find a way to pass on of her knowledge and experience to others that would follow in her footsteps. As well as embarking on this book she spent many hours working with the former Medical Director of the Bristol Cancer Help Centre, Dr Rosy Daniel, to map the work that she did for the uplift, guidance and spiritual mentorship of the clients. This allowed Rosy to create a spiritual self-development course which they called the 'Golden Path'. Pat taught this course with Rosy during the last six months of her life to twenty-four delighted students who marvelled at her lucidity and illuminated teaching; the course concluded just weeks before her death. The course also created a unique opportunity to record Pat's views in text, on film and on audio, so her great wish to pass on her experience and learning has been achieved. Her personal views can now be shared directly with those who wish to experience her inspiring truths, and receive the legacy of her teaching personally. Those wishing to take the four-weekend Golden Path course can do so by contacting Rosy's organisation, Health Creation. I know that if my mother were with us still no book about her spiritual path would be written without a deep acknowledgement of Rosy's contribution, friendship and love.

Last but by no means least, my deep thanks to all at Vala: designer Sue Gent, copy editor Kay Russell, proofreaders Iva Carrdus, Shehana Gomez, and Peter Clarke, marketer Jean Boulton, and in particular Sarah Bird. No book can come to fruition without a publishing company. No publishing company on this earth could be more perfectly in tune with its author's inner soul than Vala has been. Sarah is the essence of her company. Ethical, motivated to bring positive change to people's lives and yet gentle and steadfast in holding us all on a clear and dedicated path to publishing this book. I am sure that editing with a living author is never an easy task, but editing by committee has been a challenging stewardship, one she has managed with grace and clarity. I cannot think of Sarah without a warm smile flowing through me. My deepest thanks for taking the first and only draft of The Golden Thread and turning it into a beautiful book, a lovely legacy of my mother's spiritual path.

Felicity Biggart
February 2015

About Vala

Vala is an adventure
in community supported publishing.

We are a cooperative
bringing books to the world that explore and celebrate
the human spirit with brave and authentic
ways of thinking and being.

Books that seek to help us find our own meanings
that may lead us in new and unexpected directions.

Vala exists to bring us all into fuller relationship with our
world, ourselves, and each other.

www.valapublishers.coop/goldenthread